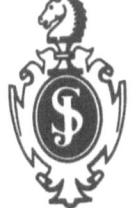

J. Beynon, G. Feifel, U. Hildebrandt
and N.J.McC. Mortensen

An Atlas
of Rectal
Endosonography

With 156 figures

Springer-Verlag
London   Berlin   Heidelberg
New York   Paris   Tokyo
Hong Kong   Barcelona   Budapest

J. Beynon, BSc, MBBS, FRCS, MS
Consultant Surgeon, Wrexham Maelor Hospital, Croesnewydd Road,
Wrexham, Clwyd, LL13 7TD, UK

G. Feifel
Professor of Surgery, Chairman, Department of General and
Abdominal Surgery, University of Saarland, Homburg, Germany

U. Hildebrandt
Professor of Surgery, Department of General and Abdominal Surgery,
University of Saarland, Homburg, Germany

N.J.McC. Mortensen, MD, FRCS
Consultant Surgeon and Clinical Lecturer, Department of Surgery and
Gastroenterology, University of Oxford Clinical Medical School, John
Radcliffe Hospital, Oxford, OX3 9DU, UK

ISBN-13:978-1-4471-1882-4   e-ISBN-13:978-1-4471-1880-0
DOI: 10.1007/978-1-4471-1880-0

British Library Cataloguing in Publication Data
An Atlas of rectal endosonography. 1. Rectum. Imaging
I. Beynon, John. 1956– 617.555

Library of Congress Cataloging-in-Publication Data
An Atlas of rectal endosonography/J. Beynon ... [et al.]
p.   cm. Includes bibliographical references.

1. Rectum—Ultrasonic imaging—Atlases. 2. Rectum—Cancer—Diagnosis—
Atlases. 3. Endoscopic ultrasonography—Atlases. I. Beynon. J. (John)
[DNLM: 1. Rectal Diseases—ultrasonography. 2. Rectal Neoplasms—
ultrasonography. WI 610 A881] RC280.R37A8 1991 616.3'507543—dc20
DNLM/DLC   91–4657
for Library of Congress   CIP

Typeset by Photo·graphics, Honiton, Devon
Printed by Henry Ling Ltd, The Dorset Press, Dorchester
28/3830-543210 Printed on acid-free paper

Foreword

It is now more than 40 years since Drs. Wild and Reid published their first experience with rectal ultrasonography from the Surgery Department at the University of Minnesota. Professor Owen H. Wangensteen, in whose laboratory the studies were carried out, recognized at that time the need for early detection in the treatment of cancer. Technical improvements over the past 20 years have made endoscopy the procedure of choice for examination of the hollow organs of the genital, urinary and gastrointestinal tracts. The simultaneous development of endosonography has had an equally dramatic impact on the practice of medicine and surgery. The technology has been demonstrated to be helpful in both benign and malignant conditions.

One of the so-called benign conditions of the anorectum is fistula-in-ano. Fistula surgery has always relied on excellent anatomic delineation of the intramuscular tracts. There is hope that adaptation of ultrasonographic technology will aid in the surgical management of this malady.

Clearly, rectal ultrasonography has considerable potential in the management of rectal carcinoma. Accuracy rates in the range of 90% for the depth of neoplastic invasion have been reported. This ability for accurate assessment will undoubtedly lead to a better definition of the population of patients that can be managed by local therapeutic means.

The proper staging of rectal neoplasms should allow a better selection of patients to be treated with other modalities such as preoperative radiation. In addition, endosonography may become the low-cost method of choice for follow-up of patients who have had restorative resections for rectal carcinoma.

There is no question that staging of rectal neoplasms will improve. Hopefully this improved clinical pathological staging

will permit more accurate comparison of data from different
institutions. This comparability of data will also permit more
multicenter trials in the management of rectal cancer.

Drs. Beynon, Feifel, Hildebrandt and Mortensen must be
congratulated on putting their pioneering efforts together in this
atlas. They have succeeded admirably in capturing the current
state of the art in this rapidly developing field. This atlas should
have interest for all who are managing patients with rectal and
perirectal disease.

April 1991   Stanley M. Goldberg, MD
                                           Clinical Professor of Surgery
                      Director, Division of Colon and Rectal Surgery
                                              Department of Surgery
                          University of Minnesota Medical School

Preface

For over a century surgeons have relied on clinical judgement and a digital rectal examination in assessing patients with rectal cancer and other anorectal disorders. With the present trend towards sphincter-saving resections, local excision in selected cases, primary or adjuvant radiotherapy and the very early work with laser therapy, there is now, more than ever before, a need for an objective method of detecting the degree of local invasion of rectal tumours. Since its introduction, endosonography has shown great potential in this area. The equipment is relatively inexpensive, can be used at the patient's couch-side, and with recent technical refinements is capable of giving brilliantly clear images of the rectal wall and surrounding tissues. The purpose of this atlas is to provide an introduction and a reference to rectal endosonographic images. We have included examples of not only the more commonplace images of normal rectal wall and rectal adenocarcinoma but examples of technical problems and rarer rectal pathology. The cases shown here are from our own experience, starting in 1984 in Homburg, and 1985 in Bristol and now Oxford.

We hope that, by using this atlas, the interpretation of rectal endosonographic images will be made more simple and the management of patients with rectal lesions before and after treatment will be improved.

Finally, thanks are due to the University of Homburg, Bristol Royal Infirmary and the John Radcliffe Hospital, Oxford, for permission to reproduce photographs. We also gratefully acknowledge the help of Gary James with some of the line illustrations.

October 1990

Neil Mortensen
John Beynon
Gernot Feifel
Ulrich Hildebrandt

Contents

1 Introduction 1

2 Clinical Staging 3

3 Radiological Staging and History 5

4 Instrumentation and Examination Technique 9

5 Anatomy 15

6 Primary Rectal Cancer 43

7 Local Recurrence 81

8 Benign Rectal Tumours, Anal Canal, Perianal Disease
   and Other Conditions 93

Appendix. TNM and pTNM Classification of Colorectal
Carcinoma 107

Bibliography 109

1 Introduction

Since the earliest days of surgery for rectal cancer, surgeons have attempted to assess the extent of local spread of the tumour before embarking on a particular operation. Digital rectal examination has always been the cornerstone of this assessment and great emphasis has been placed on the information it provided. Cooper and Edwards (1892) for example pointed out that "The height to which the growth extends, and the involvement of adjacent parts have an important bearing on the question of treatment." The subsequent introduction of sigmoidoscopy and barium examinations provided details of the luminal extent of a tumour but except in the case of very extensive tumours were not helpful in the prediction of local invasion.

With an increasing emphasis on sphincter-preserving rectal excision the question of local invasion has become the prime issue in successful treatment. Low rectal anastomoses are technically feasible but can they be achieved without compromising cancer clearance? The older argument over distal tumour clearance has been succeeded by those concerning lateral and mesorectal clearance. An ideal pre-operative staging method should be able to predict the best treatment for a particular tumour, whether that is local excision, formal major resection, or surgery with pre- or post-operative radiotherapy. This would be preferable to the most widely used current approach, which can be summarised as: remove the tumour, check the histology and then decide whether treatment has been sufficient.

2 Clinical Staging

It is surprising that the accuracy of digital rectal examination has been formally tested only in a small number of studies. In 1976, Yorke-Mason proposed a clinical staging system which he hoped would allow a more selective approach to individual tumours. He had carefully compared the physical characteristics and histology reports on resection specimens with his own pre-operative clinical assessment by digital examination. The groups he suggested were as follows.

1. *Clinical stage I (CSI)*: tumours such as benign rectal neoplasms with early invasion. These are freely mobile because the loose connective tissue space between the muscularis mucosae and the muscle coat of the rectum is not involved.

2. *Clinical stage II (CSII)*: tumours in which invasion has extended across the submucosal plane into the true muscle layer. These are therefore less mobile than CSI but without being very firmly tethered. Yorke-Mason admitted that making this fine distinction was very much a matter of experience.

3. *Clinical stage III (CSIII)*: where invasion extends through the full thickness of the rectal wall and out into the perirectal tissues there is a characteristic impression of "tethered mobility".

4. *Clinical stage IV (CSIV)*: when an adjacent structure is involved by local invasion the tumour feels fixed and immobile.

Such a clinical assessment obviously requires a great deal of experience and judgement, and this was confirmed in an elegant prospective study of 70 patients with cancer of the middle or lower third of the rectum (Nicholls et al. 1982). The two experienced specialists were most accurate in their recognition of tumours without any local spread, but were less able to distinguish between degrees of local invasion. The less experienced registrars were less accurate in the assessment of all grades of tumour. Involvement of lymph nodes assessed by palpation was detected in around 50% of cases. Tumours lying between 5 and 8 cm from the anal verge were more often treated by sphincter-saving resection when the local spread was assessed to be nil or slight, and more often by total rectal excision when it was assessed to be moderate or extensive.

So although experienced clinicians can stage tumours by digital examination with a reasonable degree of accuracy, less-experienced observers are much less accurate and upper third tumours are usually out of reach of the examining finger.

3 Radiological Staging and History of Endorectal Sonography

Radiological Staging

As new imaging techniques became available they were used to stage rectal cancer. External ultrasound scanners were particularly unsatisfactory, since the rectum is hidden within the bony pelvis and there is in any case limited resolution of gut wall because of the low frequencies used.

Computed tomography (CT) scans have been used to look at local invasion in advanced rectal cancers, with a reasonable degree of accuracy (Table 3.1) and have an undoubted place in the assessment of local recurrence, but

Table 3.1 Assessment of tumour penetration depth by computed tomography

Author	Year	Number	Accuracy (%)
Dixon et al.	1981	47	77
Thoeni et al.	1981	39	92
Zaunbauer et al.	1981	11	100
Van Waes et al.	1983	21	81
Grabbe et al.	1983	155	79
Adelsteinsson et al.	1985	94	61
Freeny et al.	1986	80	48
Thompson et al.	1986	25	79

From: Thompson et al. (1986).

early local invasion and lymph nodes are poorly demonstrated (Thompson and Calvorsen 1987).

Nuclear magnetic resonance imaging shows early promise but there is no evidence that it is any better than CT at the present time (Johnson et al. 1987a).

In view of the limitations of external ultrasound, endoluminal or intrarectal transducers have been developed and the technique and image interpretation of rectal endosonography is the subject of this book.

History of Endorectal Sonography

The first experiments with ultrasonic intraluminal scanning were made by Wild and Reid (1952, 1956). They used a rotating scanner in the rectum and compared normal rectum (Fig. 3.1) with the disturbed echo pattern changes due to cancer. In general, cancer tissue was less echogenic than normal tissue, and an example of one of their early scans is shown here (Fig. 3.2). In all they produced three working echo endoprobes and made the first observations of gut endosonography both during examinations of patients and in resected specimens in the laboratory. They hoped that their pioneering work would "inspire interest in the development of endoprobe ultrasonic techniques for the much needed detection of early localised neoplasm foci in the mucosa of the lower bowel". We now know that endoscopy has met this requirement, but the idea of using endosonography to screen for pre-symptomatic cancer was applicable to prostate carcinoma. Watanabe (1979) used a specially designed chair which placed a radial

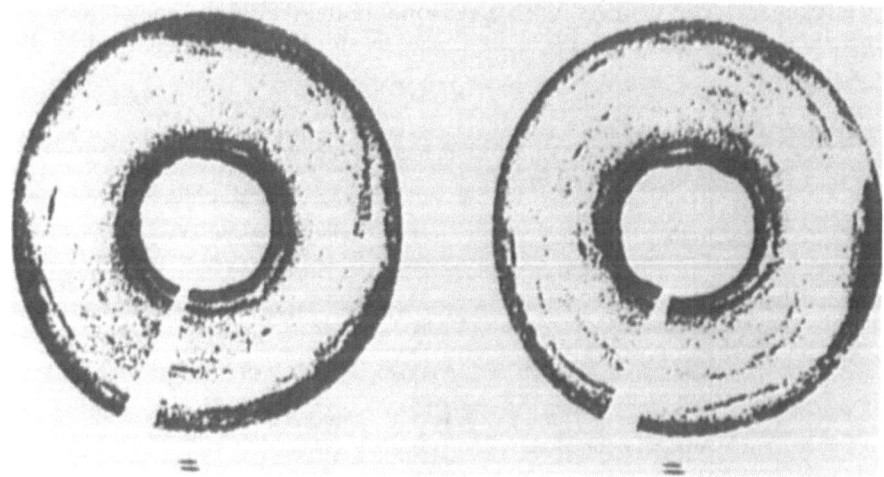

Fig. 3.1. Examples of the first sonograms of the rectum. Even here, there is a suggestion of a layered structure in the inner circular area which is the rectal wall.

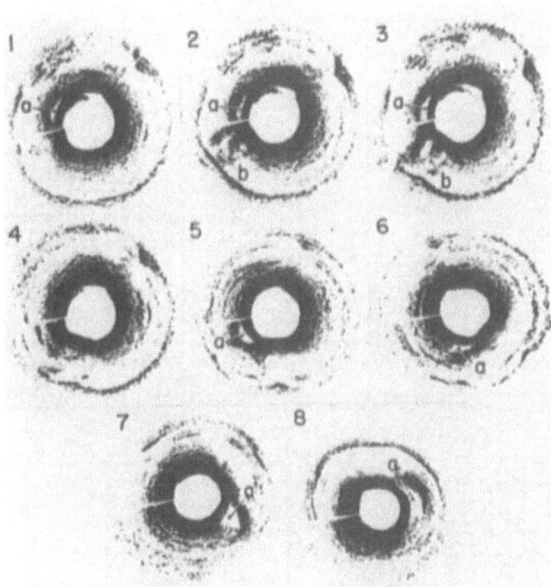

Fig. 3.2. The first demonstration of a rectal tumour using endosonography. The recurrent tumour is seen as a thickening in the rectal wall in a number of the scans (*a*). The prostate was thought to give rise to appearances at *b*.

scanner in the rectal lumen in order to "look at" the prostate. Urological endosonography equipment was then developed so that hand-held devices could be placed accurately at any position in the rectum. Alzin et al. (1983) and Dragstedt and Gamellgaard (1983) used this equipment for their early experiences of rectal cancer scanning. Since then our groups have continued to explore the advantages, disadvantages, technical hazards and interpretation problems of rectal endosonography starting with prototype 3.5 MHz transducers, then 5 MHz and now 7 MHz scanners. The images in this atlas have been collected during examinations of patients in Homburg, Bristol and Oxford since 1983. The emphasis is on the imaging of lesions already detected by other methods such as colonoscopy, but there is one area where the original aspirations of Wild and Read may yet be realised – the early detection of asymptomatic local recurrence following restorative surgery for rectal cancer.

4 Instrumentation and Examination Technique

Equipment for Endorectal Sonography

Most of the illustrations in this atlas have been taken from scans using a commercially available Bruel and Kjaer scanner type 1846 with 5 MHz and more recently 7 MHz radially scanning transducers. We have used Toshiba and Aloka linear scanning devices but have found image interpretation and manipulation of the probes within the rectum easier with the radial device. There are also a few images using a 12 MHz prototype Olympus ultrasound colonoscope.

The Bruel and Kjaer radial scanning probe is 24 cm long and 19 mm in diameter (Figs. 4.1 and 4.2) and can therefore be used in conjunction with a special 20 cm long sigmoidoscope with a minimum internal diameter of 19 mm (Fig. 4.3).

The transducer (Fig. 4.4) is fitted to the end of the rod and rotates mechanically at a rate of 4 to 6 cycles per second. The ultrasound signal is transmitted and received at 90° to the axis of the probe, and provides a 360° display of the rectum and surrounding tissues. Specifications for different types are listed in Table 4.1. A latex balloon is attached to the end of the probe over the transducer, secured by two retaining rings, and is filled with 40 to 60 ml of degassed water. The inflated balloon ensures good acoustic contact between the bowel wall and the transducer (Fig. 4.5).

Cleaning and Disinfection

The entire probe can be enclosed within a latex sheath and a small volume of gel between transducer balloon and sheath will ensure good-quality

Table 4.1. Transducer Specifications

Feature		Type 8523	Type 8539
Centre frequency	(MHz)	5.5	7.0
Focal length	(mm)	17.0	30.0
Focal range	(mm)	10–40	20–45
Axial resolution	(mm)	0.6	0.4
Beam angle to			
rotating axis	(deg.)	90	90

See also Fig. 4.4.

sonograms. Using a sheath for each examination during a series of procedures will minimise the need for cleaning. When a sheath is not used, the probe is washed in tap water, and any adherent material is gently brushed off. It should not be heated or boiled above 40°C, since the probe contains sensitive electronics and plastics. We disinfect the equipment by immersion in glutaraldehyde (Cidex) for 20 minutes at the end of a session or for 3 minutes between examinations.

Examination Technique

Position

Either the left lateral position or lithotomy position can be used, but the latter is the usual position for examination under anaesthesia for painful lesions or ultrasound-guided biopsy.

Preparation

Simple bowel preparation using a small self-administered disposable enema is usually sufficient. Where there is a great deal of faecal material in the rectum, examination is impossible and a larger enema preparation will be necessary.

Examinations are carried out with patients fully conscious and without sedation, although on occasion for very nervous subjects or those with a painful lesion intravenous midazolam and pethidine similar to that used in endoscopy will provide a comfortable procedure.

Preliminary Examination

A careful digital rectal examination is carried out first, palpating the area of interest for mobility or fixity and the presence of extra rectal lymph nodes or masses. The special 20 cm rectoscope is then passed into the rectum, the lesion inspected, biopsied if necessary, and the distance from

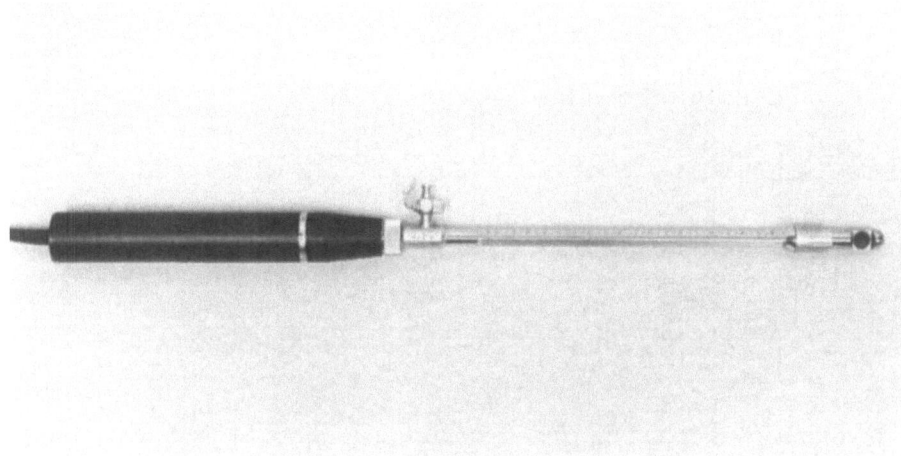

Fig. 4.1. The endoprobe used for all ultrasonic examinations: type 1850 (Bruel and Kjaer, Denmark).

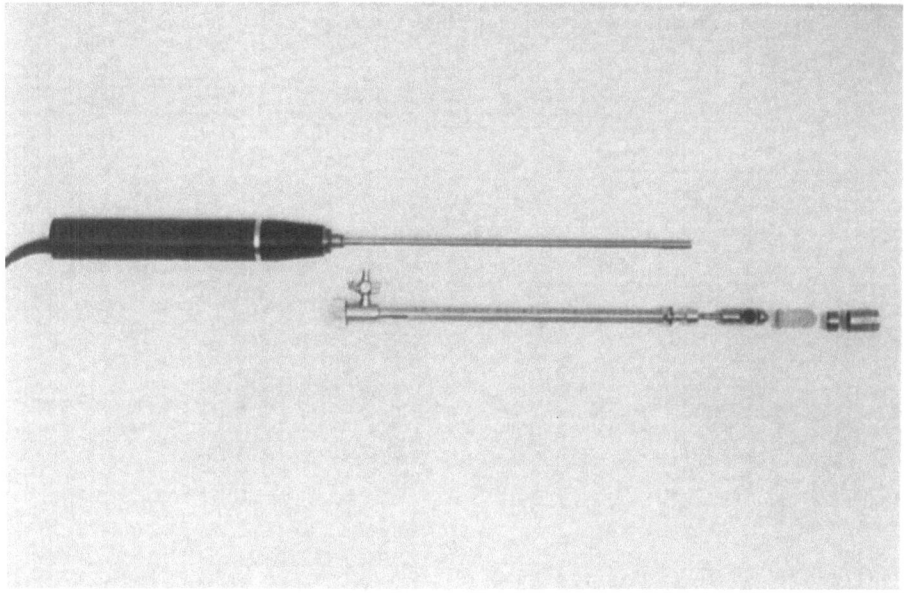

Fig. 4.2. The individual parts of the type 1850 endoprobe. These consist of rotating rod, overtube, transducer, latex balloon and retaining rings.

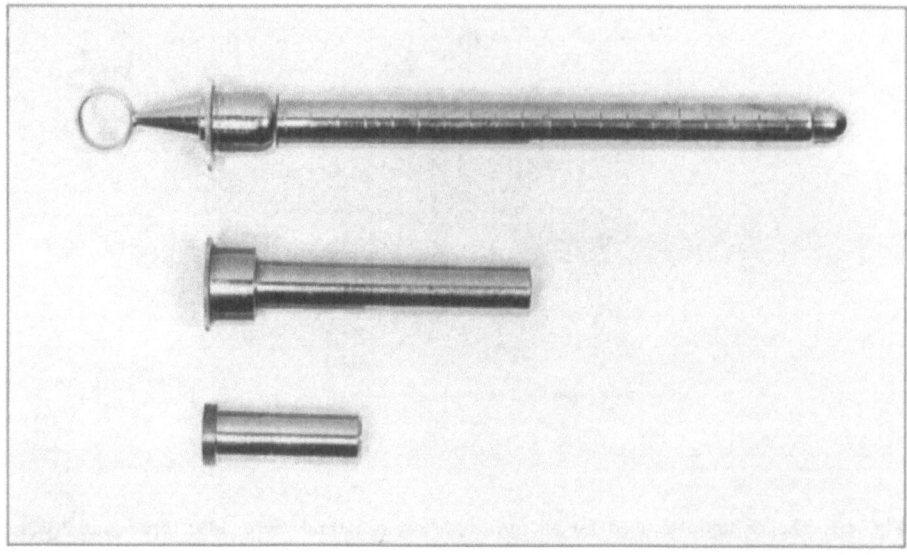

Fig. 4.3. These rectoscopes of slightly larger diameter than normal are used to position the endoprobe under direct vision when examining high or stenotic rectal tumours.

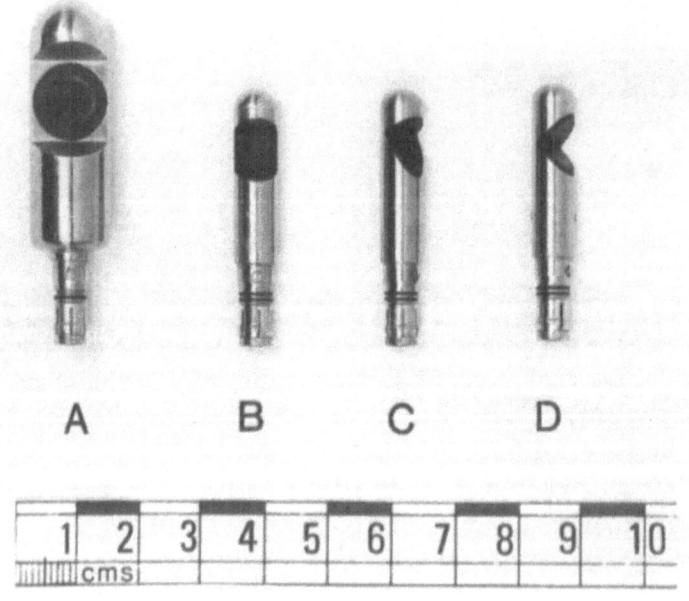

Fig. 4.4 The range of transducers used in the endosonographic examinations. These clip into the end of the rotating rod. A, 7.0 MHz 90°; B, 5.5 MHz 90°; C, 5.5 MHz 135°; D, 5.5 MHz 60°.

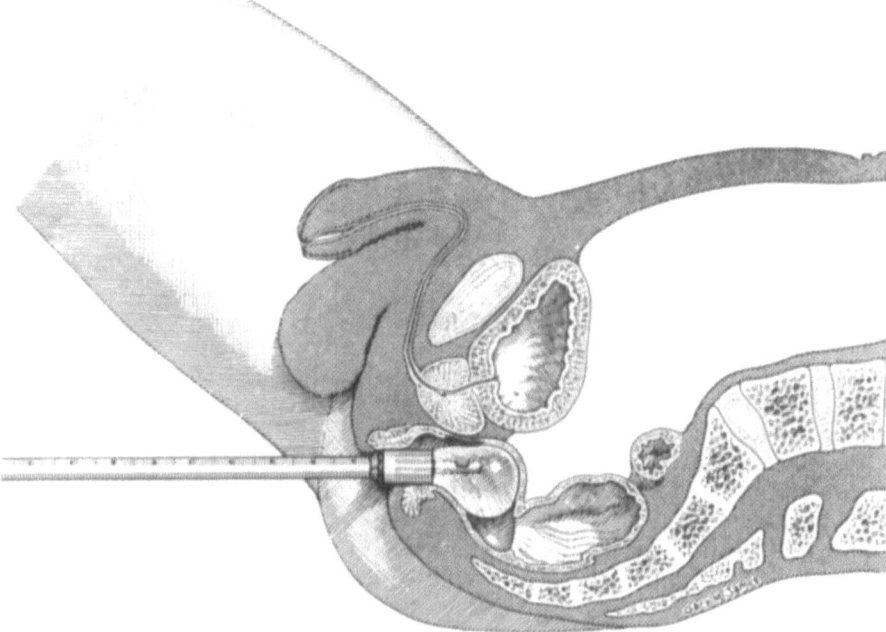

Fig. 4.5. A schematic drawing of the endoprobe within the rectum. The balloon is inflated with water to fill the rectal lumen and when scanning commences the transducer rotates inside giving a radial scan of the rectum and surrounding structures.

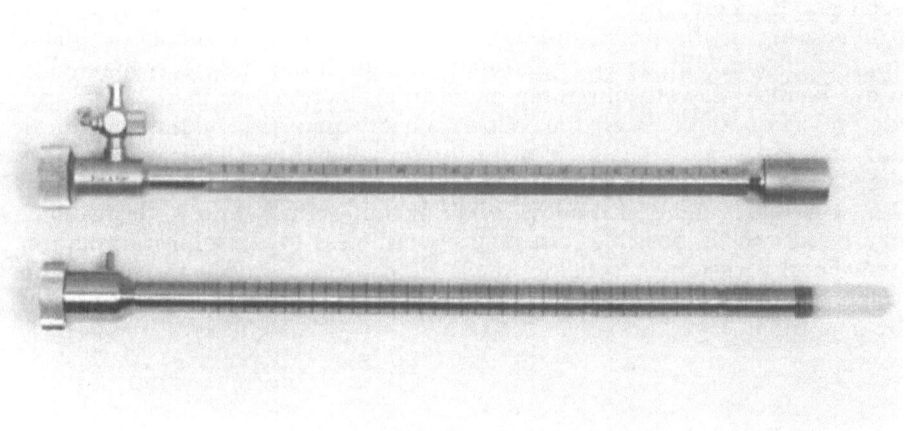

Fig. 4.6. The two overtubes used to cover the rotating rod of the type 1850 endoprobe. The tube with the plastic cap was specially designed to prevent snagging of the latex balloon by the rotating transducer when studying stenotic lesions.

the anal verge recorded. We would then usually pass the assembled endoprobe through the rectoscope above the lesion. It is possible to reach to 20 cm above the anal verge in this way, but examination in this area can be uncomfortable for the patient. The endoprobe is not usually passed blind except for very low-lying problems or when there is a low stenosis.

Rectal Endosonography

Following insertion of the probe beyond the end of the 20 cm sigmoidoscope the rubber ballon is filled with degassed water. The probe and rectoscope are then simultaneously withdrawn slowly and the transducer activated so that a 360° scan of the rectal wall and surrounding tissues is displayed on the console screen. The probe can be rocked gently backwards and forwards past areas of interest, and the volume of water in the balloon can be adjusted to bring a particular feature into the optimal focal range of the transducer. For most purposes the transducer should be positioned centrally within the lumen. Special images can be recorded for later discussion on videotape, or on a hard copy camera.

Due to distortion of the transducer balloon, the rectal wall above 12 cm cannot be rescanned without complete re-insertion of the rectoscope and scanner probe. Depending on the size and site of a lesion the examination takes between 10 and 15 minutes.

Problems Encountered During Patient Examination

Two particular limitations may be encountered when one first starts to use rectal endosonography. High rectal tumours can present problems, since manoeuvring of the probe through the lesion may be extremely difficult and there is a potential risk of perforation, though this has never happened in our hands. Very stenotic tumours with a lumen of less than 25 mm can also prove impossible, since the balloon is badly distorted and the transducer may snag. In some cases a 60° semi-forward viewing 5.5 MHz transducer (Fig. 4.4) can give useful information when positioned just below a tumour. Otherwise assessment of the lower half of the lesion with a 90° transducer may be all that is possible, but may nevertheless give useful information about local invasion. A sonolucent plastic cap can be used instead of the balloon to examine stenotic lesions but is most useful in the imaging of the anal canal (Fig. 4.6).

5 Anatomy

The Normal Sonographic Appearance of Rectal Wall

Endorectal sonography is being used to assess a wide range of abnormal rectal conditions. So that the images can be interpreted accurately, the normal sonographic anatomy must first be described.

When a 7 MHz transducer is used, the rectal wall image appears to have two hypoechoic and three hyperechoic circles (Fig. 5.1). In the centre is the transducer surrounded by the black of the water in the balloon. The first white circle represents the combination of rubber balloon, water, and mucosa interface. The middle white circle represents the interface between mucosa, submucosa and muscularis propria. Some authors have suggested that this is the interface between mucosa and submucosa, and there is continuing uncertainty over the interpretation of this layer. The outer bright circle is the interface between muscularis and fat. The inner dark circle represents the mucosa and muscularis mucosae. The outer dark circle represents the muscularis propria. Since, for example, invasion of a carcinoma into or through the muscularis propria has a major bearing on prognosis the integrity of this outer dark circle is the key to accurate reporting of cancer staging. It can be seen, however, that since there is uncertainty over the relationship between the submucosa and these endosonic layers earlier degrees of invasion are more difficult to assess.

In studies using specimens suspended in a water bath using a 7 MHz radial scanner, the balloon alone when filled with water shows as a white circle (Fig. 5.2).When the balloon is not used, the first bright circle is still present and represents the reflected waves from the surface of the mucosa. Repeating this scan with the balloon in place showed that the reflection from the balloon merged with the inner interface to produce one bright line (Fig. 5.3).

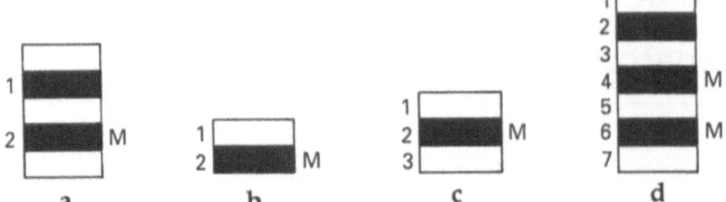

a   b   c   d

Sonographic interpretation of the rectal wall. **a** Boscaini et al. (1986), Hildebrandt et al. (1986) and Beynon et al. (1986a) describe two hypoechoic lines as real anatomical layers: 1, mucosa; 2, muscularis. **b** Rifkin and Marks (1985) interpret a hyperechoic line as mucosa (1) and a hypoechoic line as muscularis (2). **c** Konishi et al. (1985) see two hyperechoic (1, 3) and one hypoechoic (2) anatomical layer. **d** Yamashita et al. (1988) describe four hyperechoic and three hypoechoic layers. All authors agree that the outermost hypoechoic layer corresponds to the muscularis (M). (From Feifel et al. 1990, with permission.) Schematic interpretation of the sonographic appearance of the rectal wall. *T*, transducer: *I1, I2, I3*, inner, middle and outer interface; *mu*, mucosa; *mc*, muscularis propria. (From Feifel et al. 1990, with permission.)

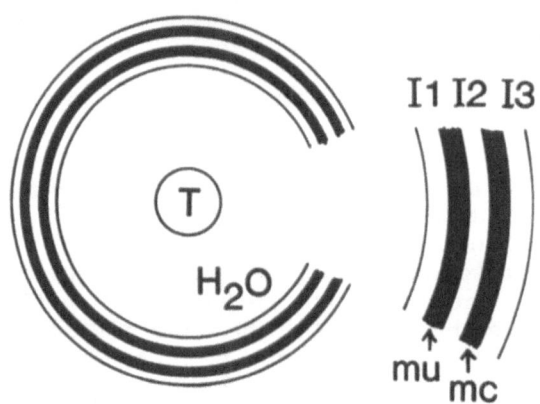

Schematic interpretation of the sonographic appearance of the rectal wall. *T*, transducer: *I1, I2, I3*, inner, middle and outer interface; *mu*, mucosa; *mc*, muscularis propria. (From Feifel et al. 1990, with permission.)

A similar method has been used to study the effects of serially removing the histological layers of the rectal wall. If the mucosa is carefully removed leaving the submucosa intact, the inner dark layer is preserved, suggesting that this layer represents an interface between mucosa and submucosa (Figs. 5.4 and 5.5). Using saline injected into the submucosa, however, the resulting plane belongs to the inner hypoechoic circle representing the mucosa. When the mucosa and submucosa are removed, the inner hypoechoic layer disappears but the outer dark layer – the muscularis propria – persists (Figs. 5.6 and 5.7).

Hildebrandt and Feifel (1986) have suggested that the sonographic appearances of the rectal wall can be explained by the following schema. A single anatomic layer has two interfaces, which appear on the sonogram as two white lines. The imaging of an anatomical layer is only possible if the axial resolution is high enough to distinguish between the transmitted and reflected ultrasound beam of the layer. Thus the layer has to have a minimum thickness corresponding to the frequency used. When a second anatomical layer has a common interface with the first, then there will be three interfaces which will correspond to three circles on the sonogram. The anatomical layers will appear as dark lines between the interfaces. In summary, if n layers have $n + 1$ interfaces, then they will be represented by $n + 1$ white circles. As far as the rectum is concerned, the two dark layers of mucosa and muscularis propria are accompanied by three white circles.

Not all the groups working with rectal ultrasound would agree with this interpretation. Rifkin in early reports described two layers. Konishi et al. (1985), using a 7.5 MHz linear scanner in vitro, have described six layers. All authors are agreed, however, that the outer hypoechoic layer corresponds to the muscularis propria. Above the peritoneal reflection this can be seen to be thickened at the site of the taenia coli (Fig. 5.8). In some cases where there is thickening or oedema of the colonic wall, the muscularis propria can be seen as two hypoechoic layers separated by a narrow bright band (Fig. 5.9). Yamashita et al. (1988) have interpreted this as the two layers of muscle – longitudinal and circular. These additional layers can also be seen in normal rectum using a 12 MHz transducer (Fig. 5.10).

Outside the muscularis propria is a hyperechoic heterogeneous mixed echo corresponding to perirectal fat, vessels and lymph nodes. Above the peritoneal reflection where the colon is covered in serosa, the serosa cannot be imaged as a separate layer. It is not usually possible to distinguish between intra- and extraperitoneal rectum, unless small-bowel images are seen alongside the rectal image.

The rectal valves of Houston are obliterated by the water-filled balloon.

Technical Factors and The Normal Sonogram

Three technical factors determine the sonographic appearance of the rectal wall.

1. The focal range of the transducer. The 7 MHz transducer has a focal range of 2 to 5 cm. Hence the individual rectal wall layers are best seen with the transducer positioned 2 to 5 cm away from the rectal wall (Fig. 5.11). This can be achieved by varying the volume of water in the balloon or by altering the axis of the probe with respect to the rectal lumen.

2. The degree of filling of the water balloon. When the balloon is filled to a large volume and pressure, the rectal wall is squeezed against the muscularis propria and this reduces rectal wall thickness (Fig. 5.12). Even if the rectal wall and transducer are within the ideal focal range, the rectal wall may not be imaged accurately due to its critical thickness. Double the amount of water is required for good images of the rectal ampulla so that it is adequately distended (Fig. 5.13).

3. The angle of the transducer with respect to the rectal wall. A transducer which is 2° or more from the ideal 90° position will transmit a beam which hits the rectal wall tangentially. As a result the appearance of the rectal wall is changed (Fig. 5.14).

Sonographic Anatomy of the Pelvis

In the male, the peritoneal reflection passes on to the posterior wall of the bladder to form the rectovesical pouch. In the female, the peritoneum passes on to the posterior fornix of the vagina to form the rectouterine pouch of Douglas. When it is filled with fluid, in appendicitis for example, the pouch and fluid can be visible on the sonogram (Figs. 5.15 and 5.16).

The Pelvic Floor

The pelvic floor, consisting of levator ani and coccygeus muscles, can be seen when the probe is placed in the upper anal canal, as a sheet extending from pelvis to coccyx (Figs. 5.17 and 5.18). At its most medial part the puborectalis can be seen passing around the back of the anorectal junction (Fig. 5.19). It is attached along the side walls of the pelvis to the obturator fascia, and the obturator internus muscle can be seen as a hypoechoic band in front of the hyperechoic reflection from the symphysis pubis (Fig. 5.19).

Within the anal canal, the balloon cannot be inflated far enough to bring the sphincter muscles into focus. However, using only a little inflation or a plastic cap over the transducer, the internal sphincter is more hypoechoic than the external sphincter. The mucosa is a hyperechoic layer (Fig. 5.20).

The Male (Fig 5.21)

The sonographic appearance of the bladder depends on the amount of liquid within it (Fig. 5.22). When empty it is thick walled and irregular. The prostate has a clear outer edge and a homogeneous hypoechoic pattern (Fig. 5.23). Flecks of calcification giving a bright echo are common. The rectovesical fascia of Denonvilliers passes between rectum and prostate and is an important surgical plane in pelvic dissection. The clear edge of prostate and this plane are important in the assessment of an anterior rectal cancer and its potential local invasion into the prostate (Figs. 5.24 and 5.25). Above the prostate are the seminal vesicles, and these are hypoechoic and of varying size (Fig. 5.26). Just below the prostate the bulbourethral glands can be identified on either side of the bulbar urethra (Fig. 5.27).

The Female (Fig. 5.28)

Anterior to the rectum is the vagina, separated from it by the rectovaginal septum (Fig. 5.29). The vagina is seen as a dark horizontal ellipse with a hyperechoic wall. Tumours penetrating the anterior rectal wall into the septum or vagina can be seen clearly. The uterus has a sharp border and is usually easily seen (Figs. 5.30, 5.31 and 5.32) but the ovaries (Figs. 5.33 and 5.34) and tubes (Fig. 5.35) are less consistently imaged on account of size, position or age of the patient.

The Vessels

The superior rectal artery (Fig. 5.36), a branch of the inferior mesenteric artery, can sometimes be seen on a sonogram. It divides at the level of S3 into two branches passing down on either side of the rectum. The middle and inferior rectal arteries cannot usually be located accurately. The rectal veins anastomose freely.

Blood vessels are hypoechoic and have a bright reflection of the echo at their edge. Veins can be distinguished from arteries by their appearance in different planes, running in and out of the sonogram as the probe is moved. Arteries by contrast run parallel with the rectum and are usually cut in transverse section.

The iliac arteries can be occasionally imaged up to the bifurcation (Fig. 5.37).

The branching continuous characteristics of hypoechoic vessels are the criteria used to distinguish them from hypoechoic lymph nodes (Fig. 5.38).

Lymph Nodes

Lymphatics from the area above the dentate line in the anal canal drain into mesorectal and internal iliac lymph nodes, and on to nodes along the superior rectal artery, the inferior mesenteric artery and eventually nodes along the aorta.

In the normal mesorectum, normal lymph nodes are rarely greater than 3 mm in diameter and the number of nodes ranges from 8 to over 20. Since they have an echo pattern similar to that of fat, they are not usually imaged even with high frequency transducers. The appearance of enlarged lymph nodes will be discussed later.

Artefacts

There are a number of technical problems which may spoil the quality of a normal sonogram. Air bubbles in the water-filled balloon cast multiple bright echoes which may obscure mural detail (Fig. 5.39). Solid faeces in the rectum cast an echo shadow which completely obscures the underlying structures (Figs. 5.40 and 5.41).

Reverberation of ultrasound signals casts a series of concentric rings, but it is usually possible to see the sonogram clearly otherwise (Fig. 5.42).

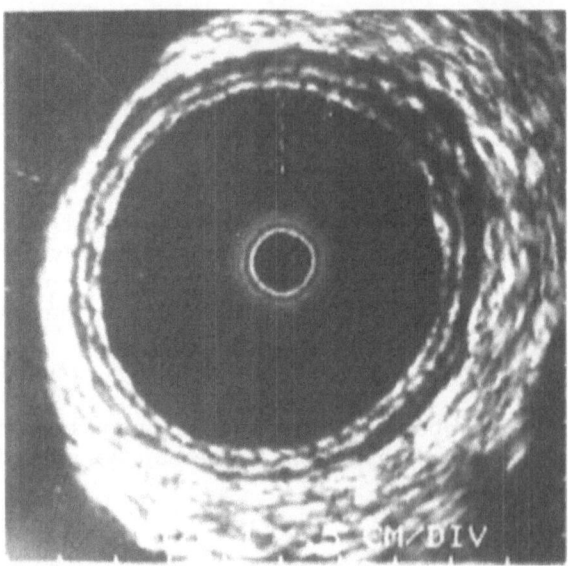

Fig. 5.1. An ultrasonic scan of an intact rectal specimen suspended in a water bath. Five distinct ultrasonic layers are seen.

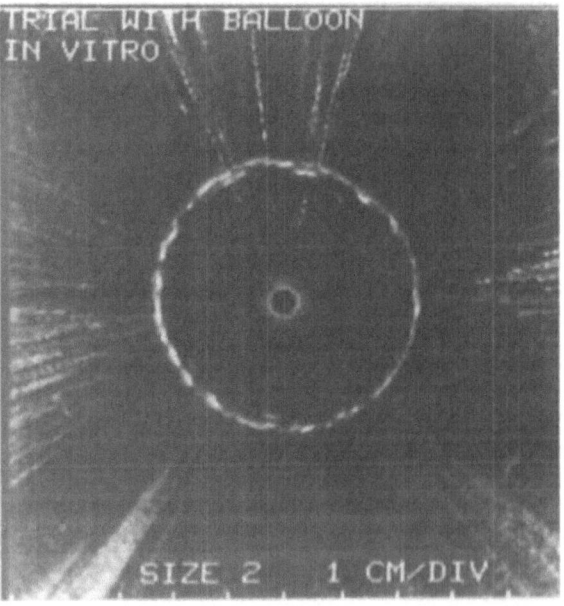

Fig. 5.2. An ultrasound scan performed with just the balloon surrounding the transducer. The balloon produces an echogenic signal of its own.

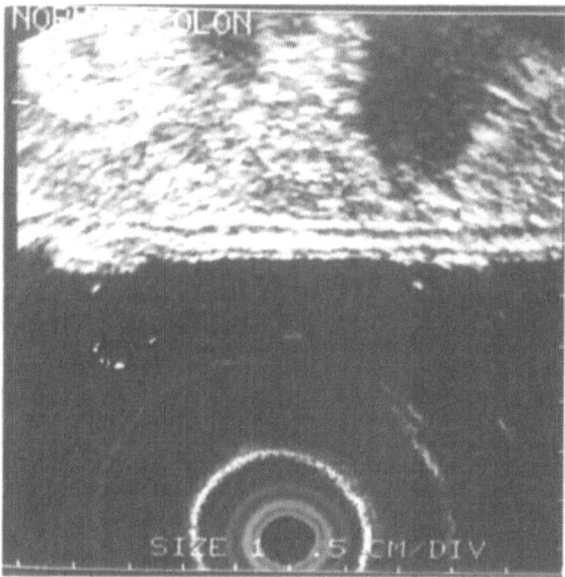

Fig. 5.3. In this scan the balloon has been interposed between the transducer and the specimen. No alterations of the five-layered image produced by the bowel wall is seen.

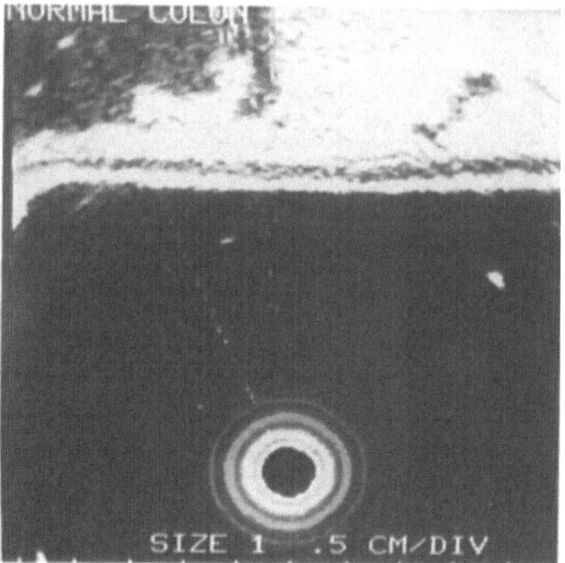

Fig. 5.4. A scan of a specimen following the removal of the mucosa and muscularis mucosae. Three layers are now imaged which correspond histologically to submucosa, muscularis propria and perirectal fat.

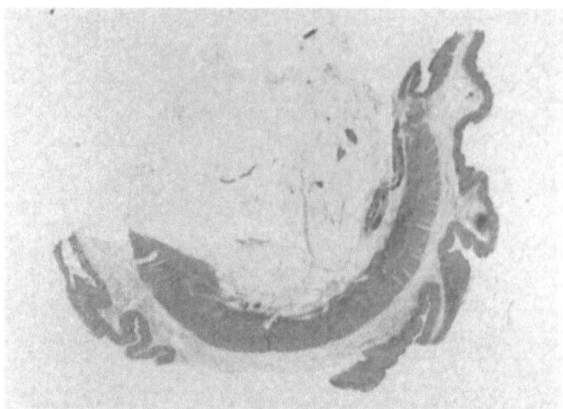

Fig. 5.5. A histological section from the specimen scanned in Fig. 5.4. This shows the histological layers left after removal of the mucosa and muscularis mucosae.

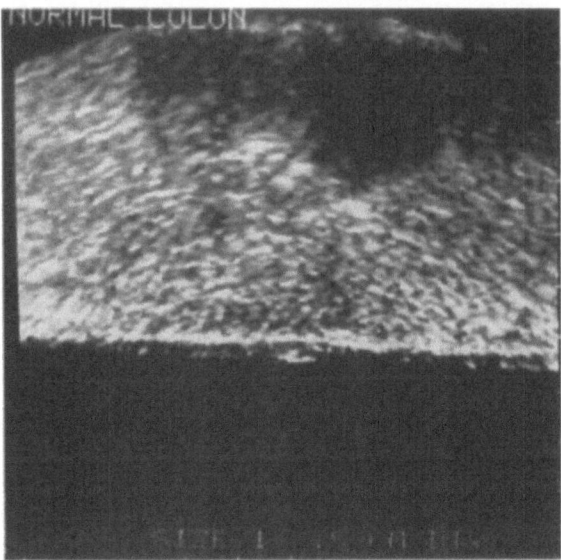

Fig. 5.6. A scan of a specimen following removal of the mucosa, muscularis mucosae and submucosa. Two ultrasonic layers were imaged.

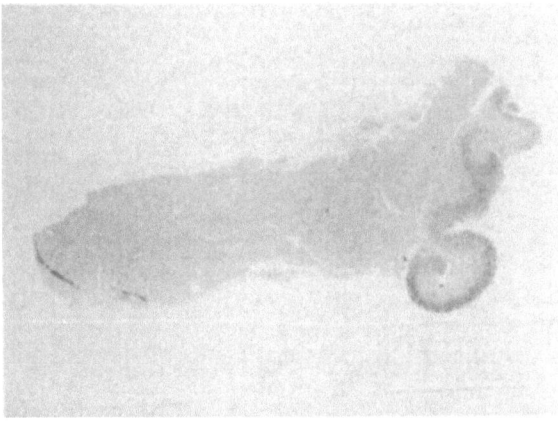

Fig. 5.7. The histological section of the specimen imaged in Fig. 5.6. Only the muscularis propria and perirectal fat remain.

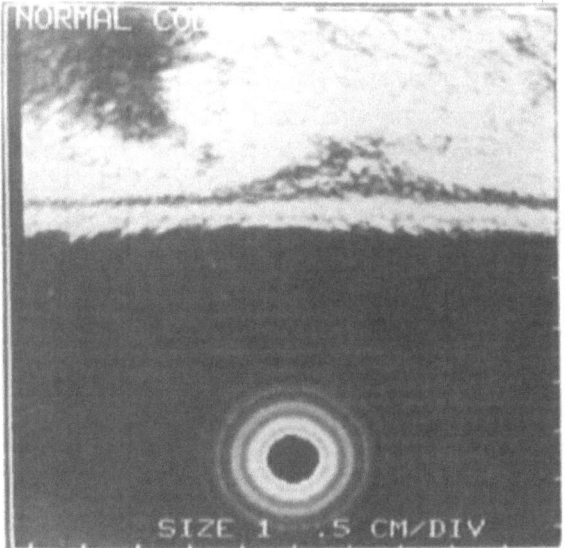

Fig. 5.8. An ultrasonic examination of a colonic specimen suspended in a water bath. Five layers are clearly displayed and also a thickening in the fourth hypoechoic layer of muscularis propria which is the taenia coli.

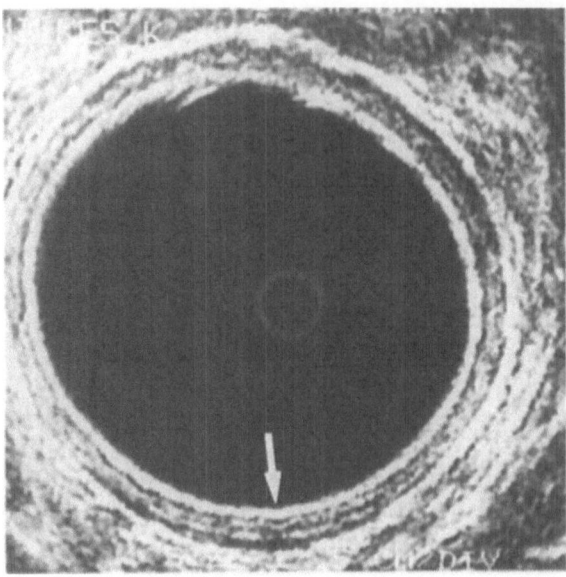

Fig. 5.9. An examination of a normal patient's rectum showing again a five-layered image. However, in the 6 o'clock position (*arrowed*) seven layers are seen.

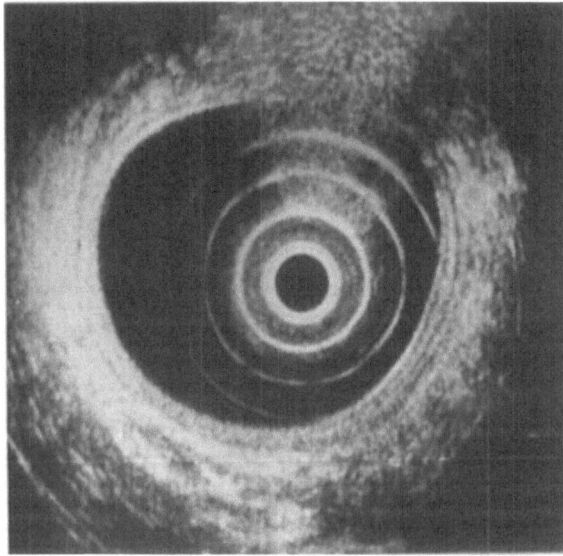

Fig. 5.10. With 12 MHz transducer, Olympus ultrasound colonoscope. Note the characteristic artefact echoes within the water-filled balloon. In the bottom right-hand corner as many as seven or nine layers can be seen in normal rectal wall.

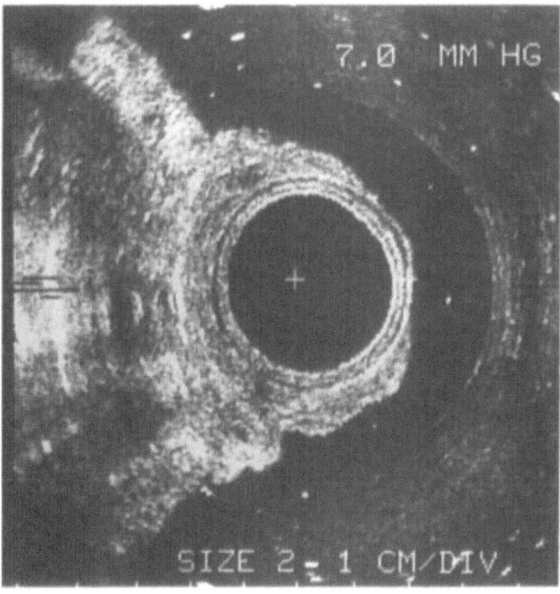

Fig. 5.11. Ideal situation: transducer in focal length (2 to 5 cm), not too much water, not squeezing the layers.

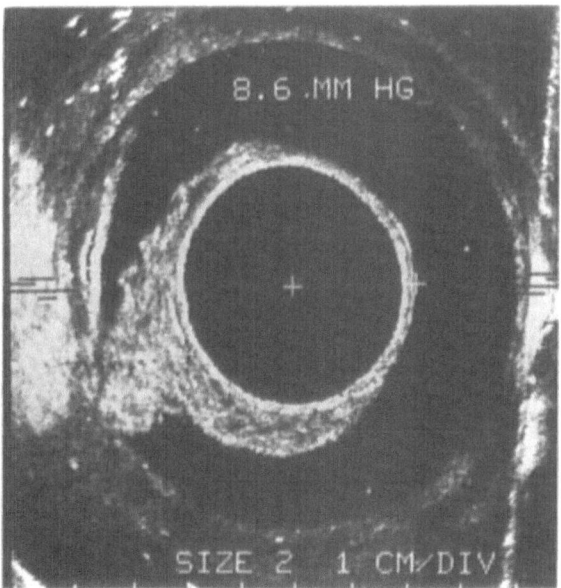

Fig. 5.12. Water bath study of normal rectal wall. Correlation of intraballoon pressure (8.6 mmHg (approx. 11.5 pa)) focal length (2.7 cm) and visualisation of the layers. The rectal wall is in the focal length of the transducer (2 to 5 cm) but due to the maximal filling of the balloon the layers of the rectal wall are squeezed and therefore the different layers are not discernible.

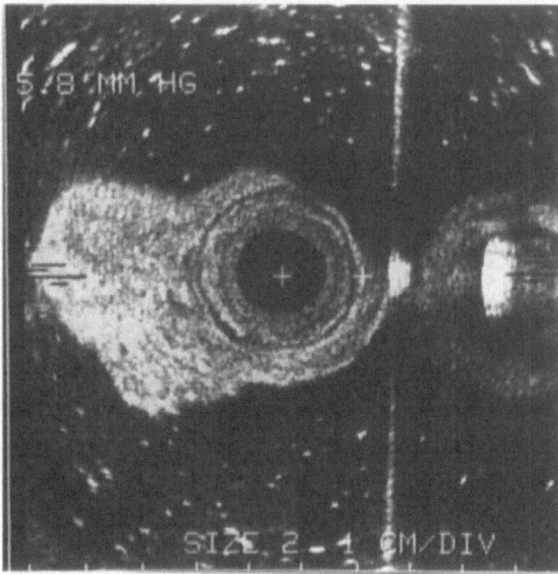

Fig. 5.13. Not enough water in the balloon, not the ideal position of the transducer (1.2 cm). For these two reasons (no distention of the rectal wall, transducer not in ideal position) there is merging of the layers.

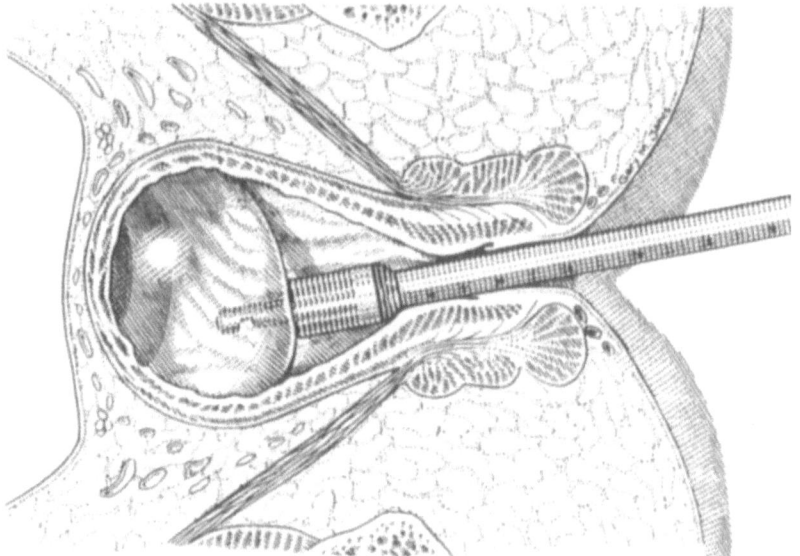

Fig. 5.14. If the probe is high in the rectum and not vertical as shown in this diagram then a true transverse section through the rectal wall may result on one side of the scan while a longitudinal section along the length of the bowel is seen on the other.

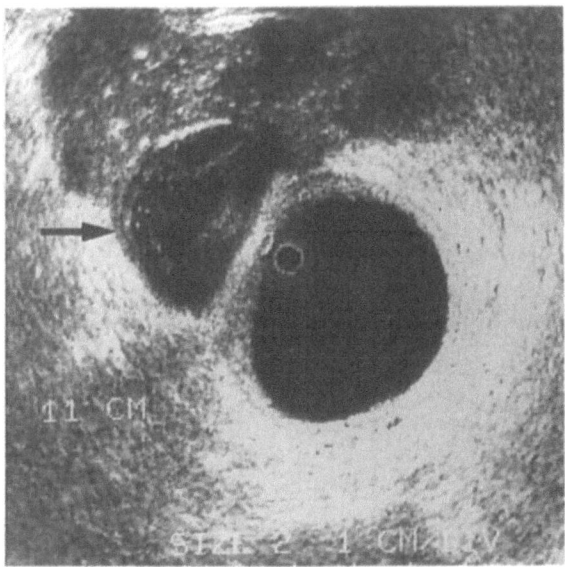

Fig. 5.15. Fluid in the pouch of Douglas (*arrow*) in a patient with perforated appendix.

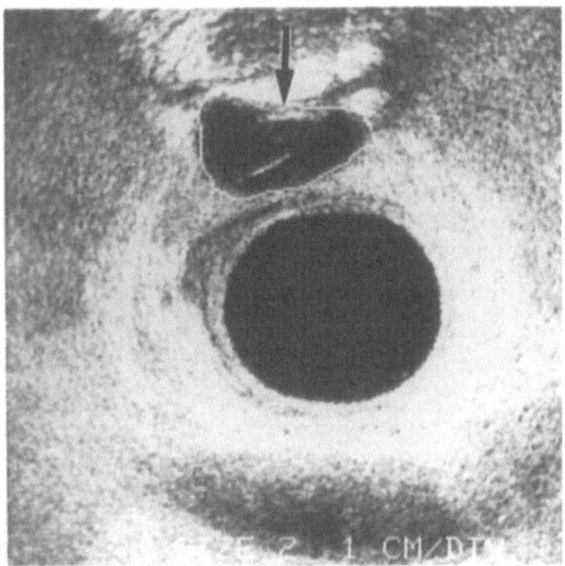

Fig. 5.16 Fluid in the pouch of Douglas (*arrow*) post-operatively: fever, white blood cells elevated.

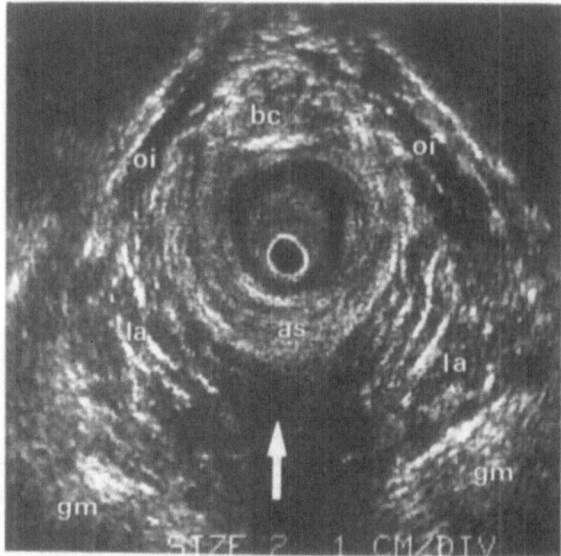

Fig. 5.17. Male pelvic floor. Note the anal sphincter (*as*), and bulbocavernosus (*bc*) muscle around the urethra. The muscles of the pelvic floor are obturator internus (*oi*) and levator ani (*la*). Note gluteus maximus (*gm*). The *arrow* marks the hypoechoic area, i.e. the space between the buttocks.

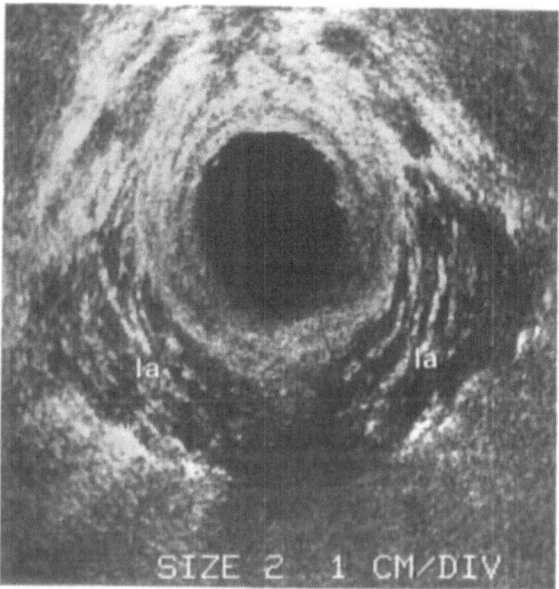

Fig. 5.18. Pelvic floor showing levator ani muscle (*la*) behind the rectum.

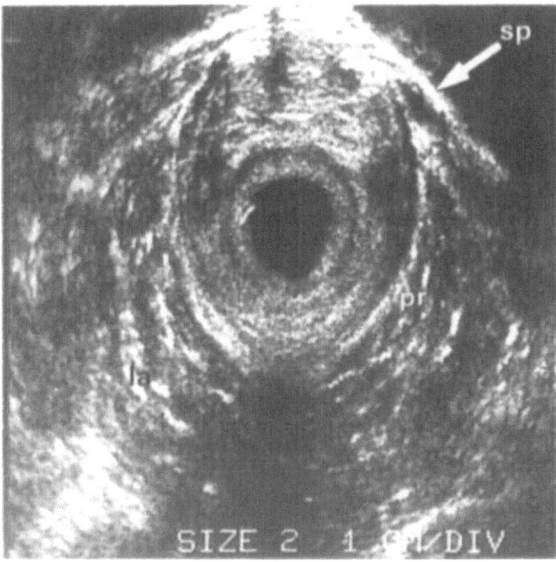

Fig. 5.19. Female pelvic floor. Note puborectalis muscle (*pr*) passing around the back of the anal canal. The introitus of the vagina (*v*) is anterior; the symphysis pubis (*sp*) and levator ani (*la*) can be seen more laterally.

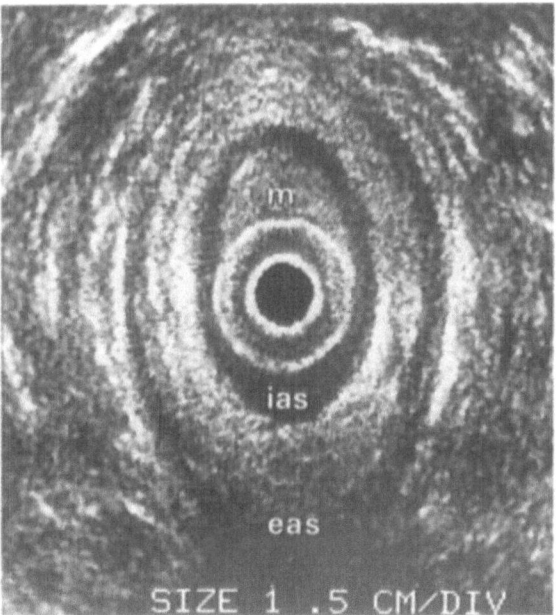

Fig. 5.20. Anal canal. Inner hyperechoic circle: mucosa (*m*). Inner hypoechoic circle: internal anal sphincter (*ias*). Next hyperechoic: external anal sphincter (*eas*) together with longitudinal conjoint muscle.

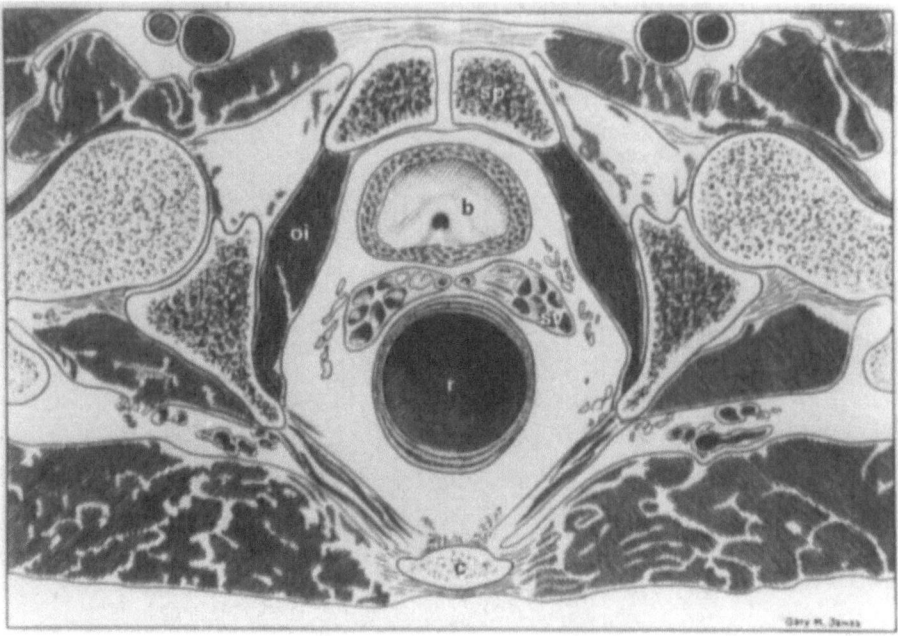

Fig. 5.21. Schematic representation of the male pelvis in transverse section at the level of the seminal vesicles (*sv*) to illustrate the structures which might be imaged ultrasonically at this level. *b*, bladder; *r*, rectum; *oi*, obturator internus; *c*, coccyx; *sp*, symphysis pubis.

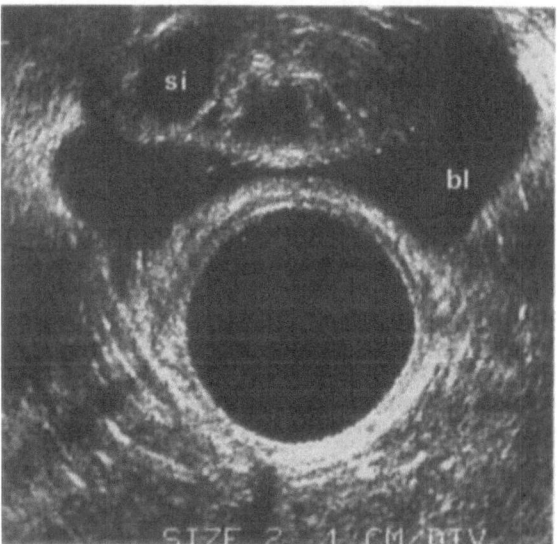

Fig. 5.22. Partly emptied bladder (*bl*) with small intestine (*si*) loops on the roof of the bladder.

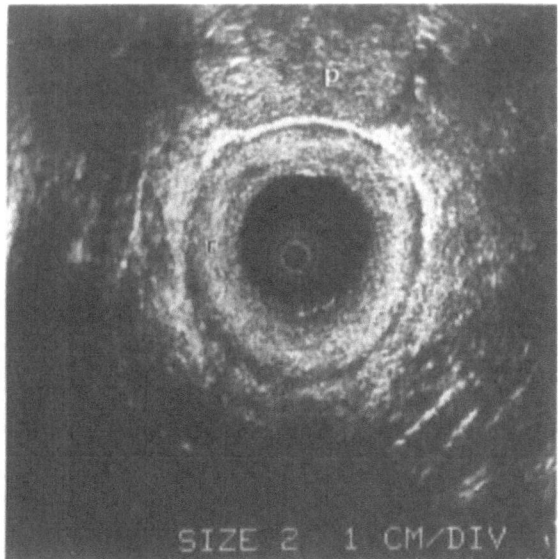

a

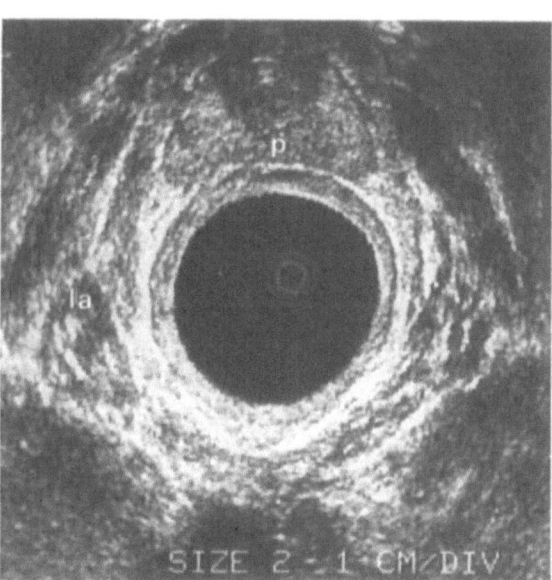

b

Fig. 5.23. a The prostate (*p*), with a clear plane separating if from the lower rectum (*r*), thick walled here because it is cut tangentially. **b** The prostate (*p*) at a lower level. *la*, levator ani.

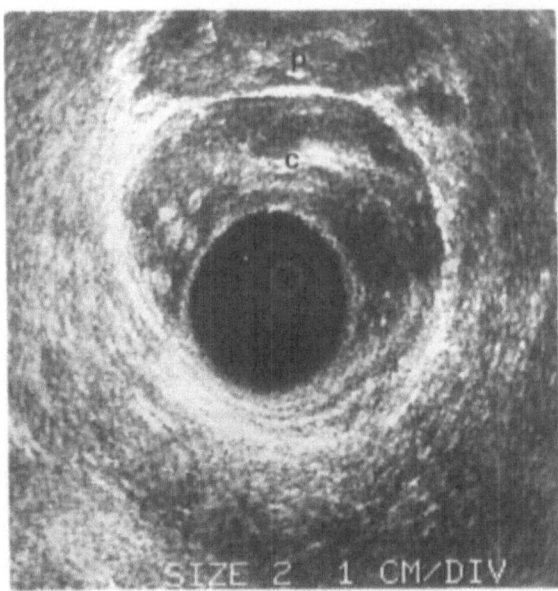

Fig. 5.24. Semicircular rectal cancer (*c*) at anterior rectal wall. No penetration into prostate (*p*).

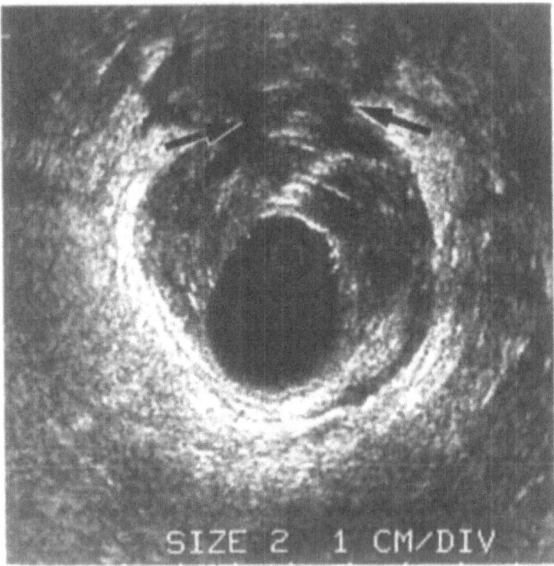

Fig. 5.25. Same patient as in Fig. 5.24, same tumour where the tumour penetrates into prostate (*arrow*).

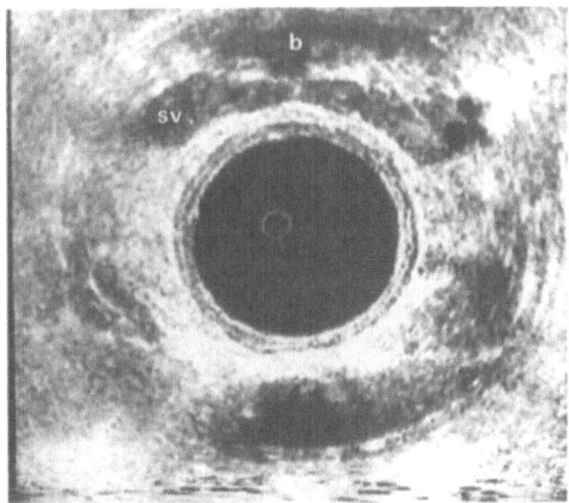

Fig. 5.26. The seminal vesicles (*sv*) and bladder (*b*).

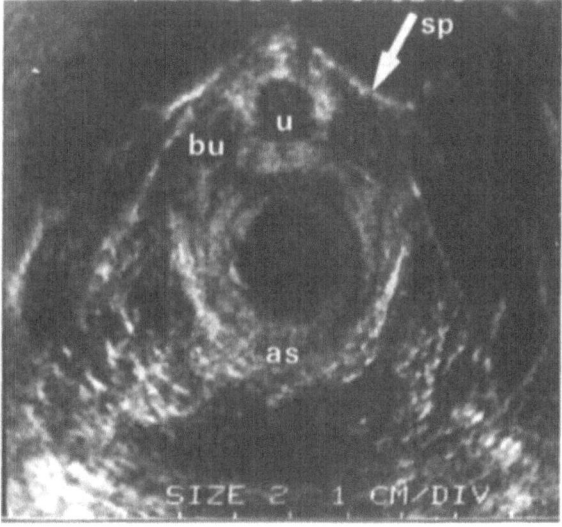

Fig. 5.27. Male pelvis. Anteriorly is the bulbar urethrar (*u*) and on either side the bulbourethral glands (*bu*). *as*, anal sphincter; *sp*, symphysis pubis.

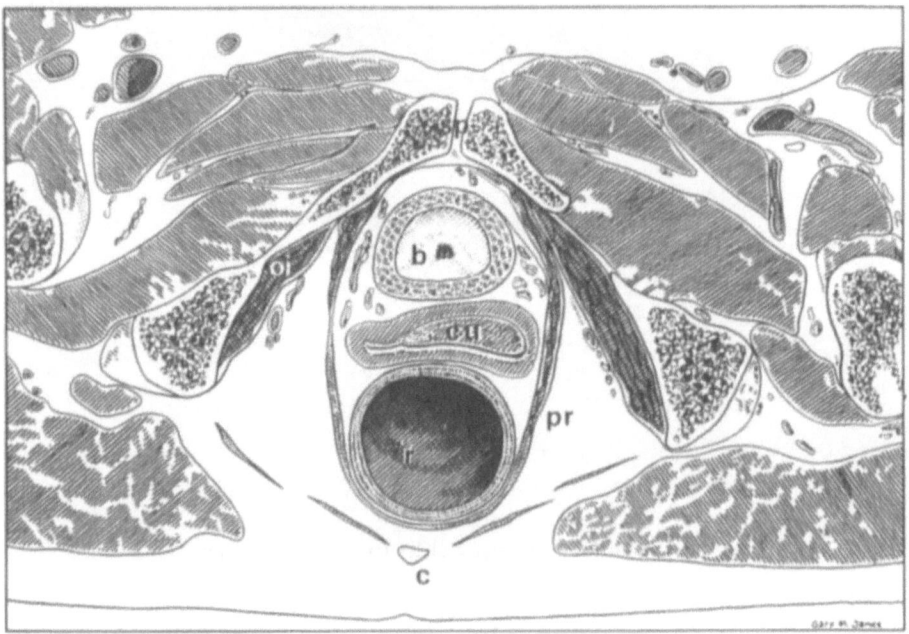

Fig. 5.28. Drawing of the female pelvis in transverse section at the level of the cervix uteri (*cu*) to illustrate the structures which might be imaged ultrasonically at that level. *b*, bladder; *r*, rectum; *sp*, symphysis pubis; *c*, coccyx; *pr*, puborectalis; *oi*, obturator internus.

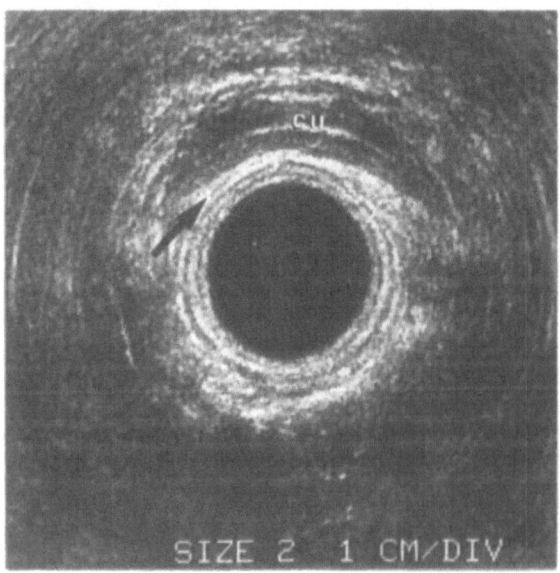

Fig. 5.29. Cervix of uterus (*cu*) and rectovaginal septum (*arrow*).

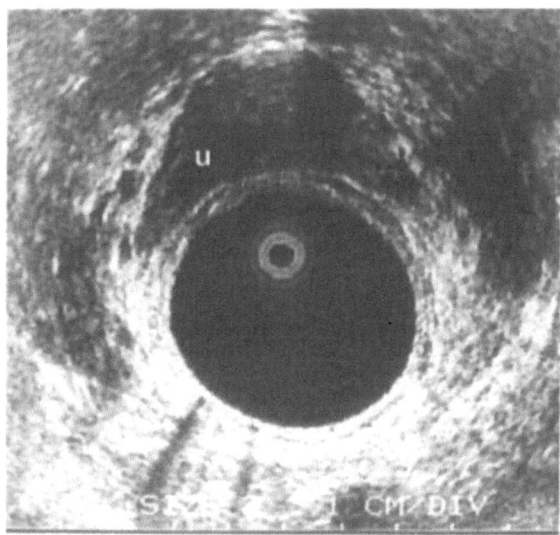

Fig. 5.30. The uterus (*u*) has a clear edge.

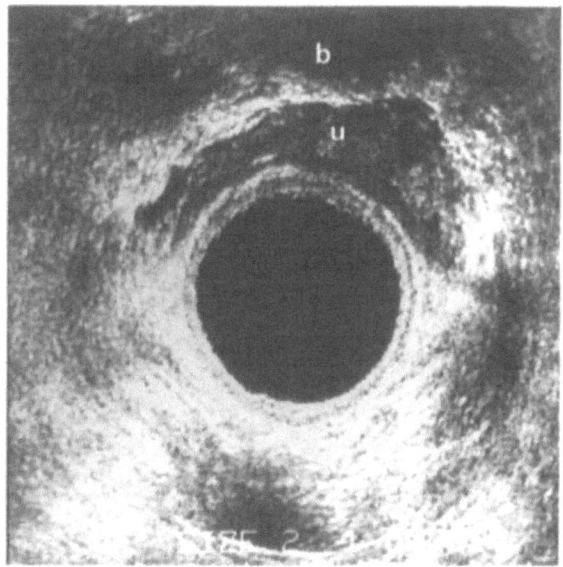

Fig. 5.31. The uterus (*u*) at a higher level, with the bladder (*b*) anteriorly.

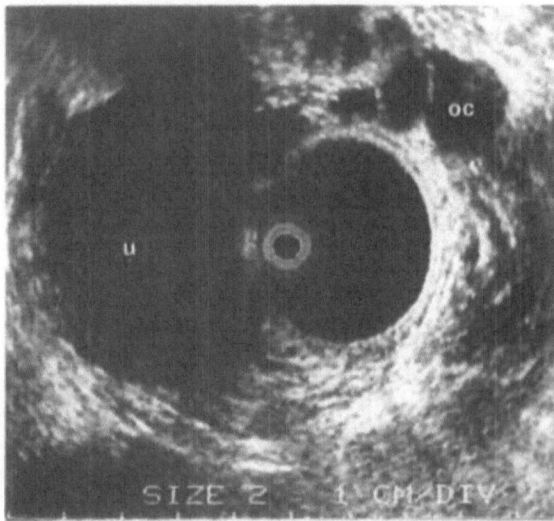

Fig. 5.32. In this patient the uterus (*u*) has moved to the right side following an anterior resection and is seen as a large hypoechoic area to the left of the scan. An ovarian cyst (*oc*) is lying anterior to the rectum.

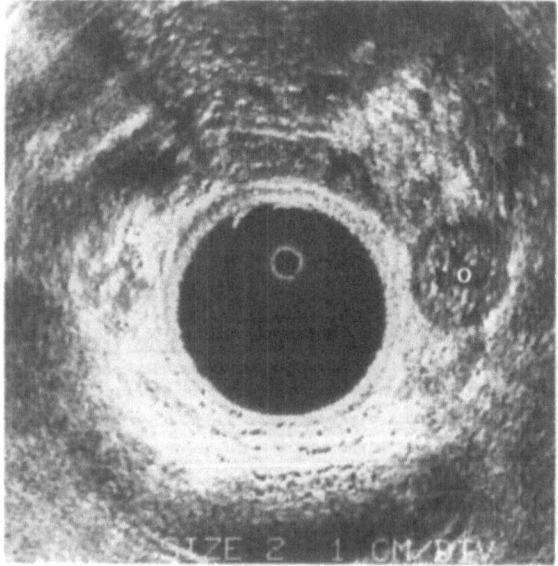

Fig. 5.33. Left ovary (*o*).

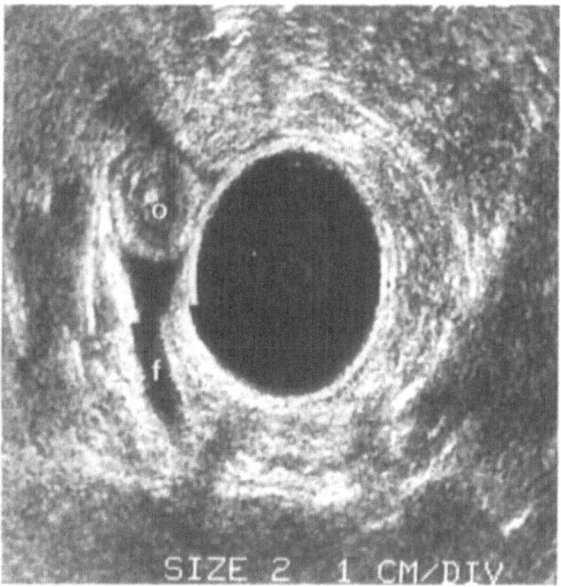

Fig. 5.34. Right ovary (*o*). Beneath it is a small collection of free peritoneal fluid (*f*).

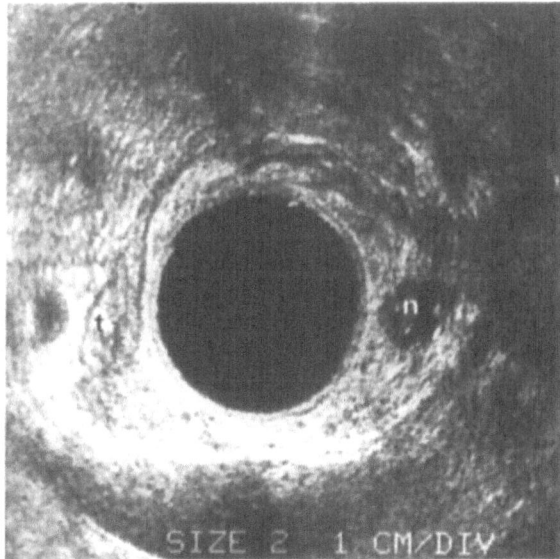

Fig. 5.35. Ovarian tube (*t*). Adjacent to the rectum is a hypoechoic lymph node metastasis (*n*).

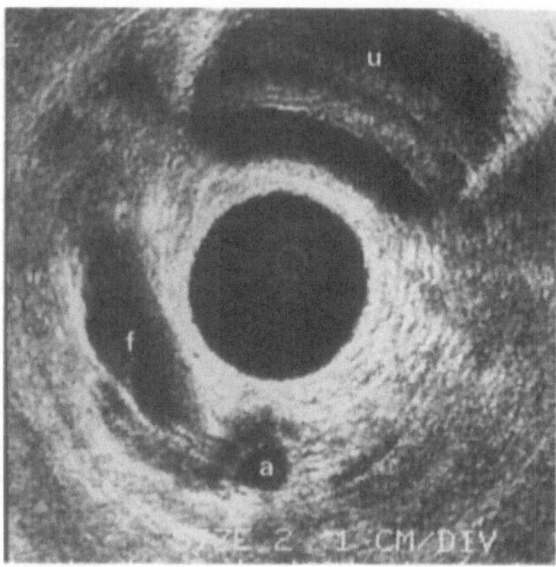

Fig. 5.36. Superior rectal artery (*a*). There is free fluid (*f*) in the pelvis, and the uterus (*u*) is anteverted and seen anterior to the empty bladder.

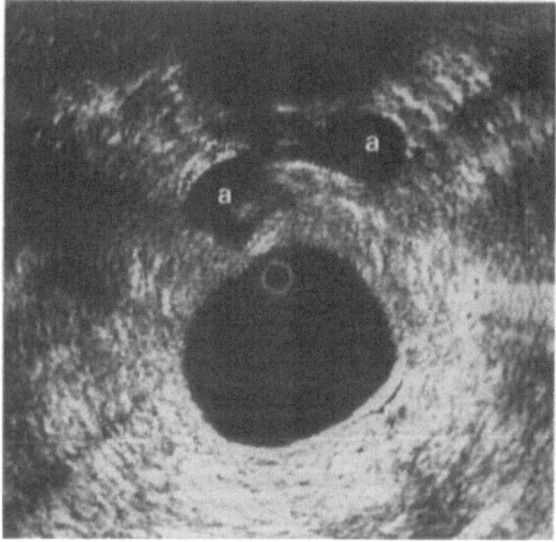

Fig. 5.37. Iliac arteries (*a*) near the bifurcation, at the sacral promontory.

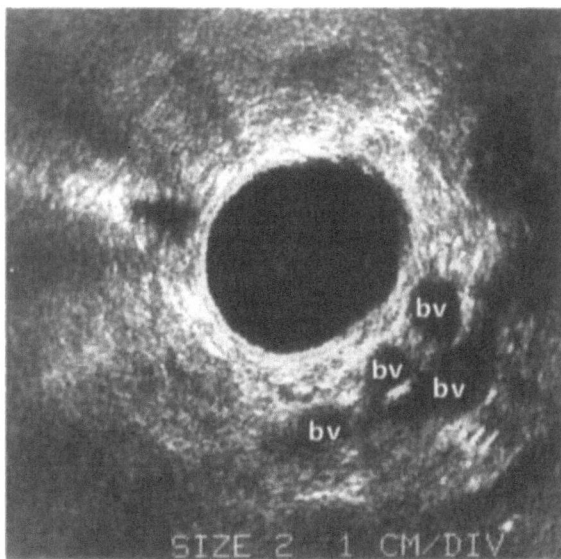

Fig. 5.38. Iliac arteries and veins, but it is not possible to distinguish between them on this sonogram. *bv*, blood vessels.

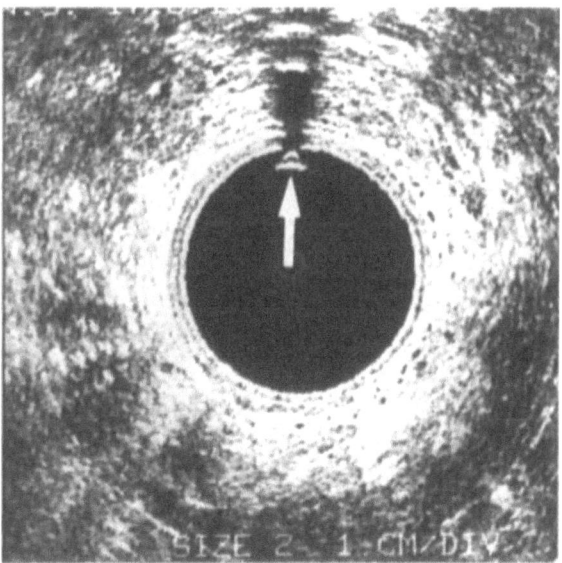

Fig. 5.39. Artefact: shadow due to air bubble (*arrow*).

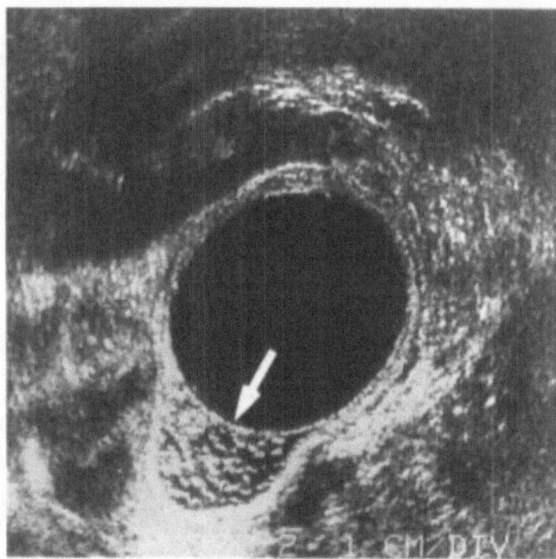

Fig. 5.40. Artefact: faeces between balloon and rectal wall
– characteristic hyperechoic spots (*arrow*).

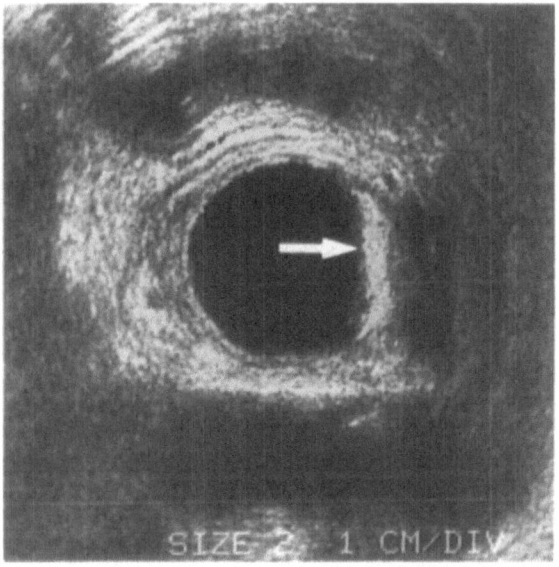

Fig. 5.41. Artefact: faeces between balloon and rectal wall
mucosa, causing hyperechoic reflection (*arrow*).

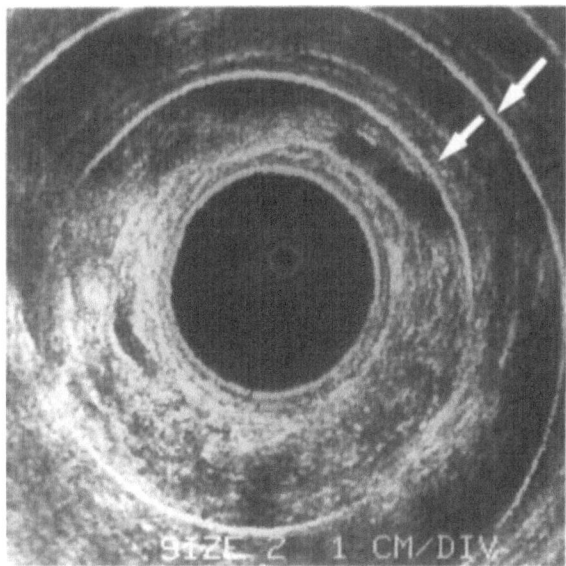

Fig. 5.42. Artefact: reflections of the first echo (*arrows*).

6 Primary Rectal Cancer and Local Invasion

Assessment of Tumour Penetration Depth

Rectal cancer has a hypoechoic apearance on the sonogram, and, as it invades deeper through the rectal wall, the normal sonographic anatomy is disrupted. The accuracy of endosonography for diagnosing rectal cancers is given for some authors in Table 6.1. By comparing the changes caused by a tumour with the normal sonogram the depth of tumour invasion can be assessed. So that this invasion can be reported in a standardised way it has been compared to histopathological staging methods. The Dukes classification has the disadvantage that a Dukes B cancer may also be a tumour invading the mesorectum early or one with wide local invasion. The UICC (Union Internationale Contre Le Cancer) TNM (tumour–node–metastasis) system (see Appendix), though not so widely used is more

Table. 6.1. Accuracy of endosonography for rectal cancer

Author	Year	Number	Correct	Accuracy (%)
Dragstedt and Gammelgaard	1983	13	11	85
Hildebrandt and Feifel	1985	25	23	92
Konishi et al.				
Linear scan	1985	38	32	84
Radial scan	1985	23	10	43
Romano et al.	1985	23	21	91
Saitoh et al.	1986	88	79	90
Hildebrandt et al.	1986	76	67	88
Rifkin and Wechsler	1986	81	68	84
Beynon et al.	1986e	67	61	91
Beynon et al.	1987b	100	93	93

precise for tumour invasion subdividing transmural invasion into three rather than just two groups (Fig. 6.1). Examples of each of these are shown here. The prefix is as first suggested by Hildebrandt and Feifel (1985) has been adopted.

uT1 (Figs. 6.2 to 6.8)

This is a tumour confined to the mucosa and submucosa. It does not interrupt the middle bright interface. The distinction between a benign uT0 lesion and an early uT1 is very difficult to make.

uT2 (Figs. 6.9 to 6.19)

Here, the tumour is confined to the rectal wall. On the sonogram a uT2 tumour does not interrupt the outer surface. The dark hypoechoic band corresponding to muscularis propria may be distorted or thinned but the outer echo is still intact.

uT3 (Figs. 6.20 to 6.30)

The tumour penetrates through the rectal wall and its perirectal fat. Here the sonogram shows interruption and disruption of the outer interface. This may happen at only one point of a tumour so that scanning backwards and forwards across the thickest part of the tumour has to be carried out very carefully to identify the breach in the outer echo. Direct infiltration into the vagina, uterus, bladder and prostate can occur. The plane between the anterior wall of the rectum and the prostate corresponding to the fascia of Denonvilliers has been described above. When this is intact there is no infiltration of the prostate. Similarly anterior tumours in female patients can be assessed for direct involvement of the vagina. Occasionally a bulky tumour may perforate, with abscess formation, and this gives the appearance of a dark anechoic area similar to the water in the balloon (Fig. 6.30).

uT4 (Figs. 6.31 to 6.35)

The tumour invades surrounding organs giving local fixation.

Understaging and Overstaging

It is important to emphasise that the best results are obtained using a 7 MHz transducer. In our earlier experience with lower frequency (3.5 and 5.0 MHz) transducers the different layers were not imaged with enough clarity to give a sharp edge to the tumour.

Minor degrees of invasion assessed histologically as 1 or 2 mm extensions into muscle or mesorectal fat are impossible to predict by endosonography and are the main cause of understaging.

In our series there is a greater tendency to overstage as uT3 rather than underestimate a lesion. This is clinically relevant, since overstaging will not result in undertreatment.

The final reason for error is technical. Unless the area of interest is within the focal range of the 7 MHz transducer (2 to 5 cm) and is hit at a 90° angle distortion may occur. This is especially important just inside the rectal ampulla where the optimal 90° angle of incidence is difficult to achieve (see Fig. 6.28).

Lymph Node Metastases (Figs. 6.36 to 6.65)

Lymph nodes are best seen with the 7 MHz transducer. Normal lymph nodes less than 3 mm in diameter have an echo pattern similar to that of mesorectal fat and are not usually seen. Obviously mesorectal nodes are the easiest to scan and nodes high up the mesenteric artery cannot be imaged. Less than 50% of the nodes seen by a pathologist in a resection specimen are seen by ultrasound.

Enlarged lymph nodes can result from non-specific inflammation or metastasis.

Inflammatory lymph nodes are 4 mm or more in diameter. They are normally hyperechoic (Figs. 6.45 and 6.46) and may be separated from the surrounding fat by a thin hypoechoic circle, but their margin is usually indistinct. They have a homogeneous pattern which is a little less echogenic than the surrounding fat.

Metastatic lymph nodes have a hypoechoic appearance and are usually 4 mm or more in diameter. An irregular hypoechoic pattern similar to, or more hypoechoic than, the primary tumour, together with a sharp border, is highly suggestive of malignancy. However, some hypoechoic nodes are inflammatory and not metastatic. Circumscribed hypoechoic areas can also be due to islands of tumour outside the rectal wall but not in nodes. Blood vessels in cross-section may also give rise to a false positive diagnosis.

Using these criteria and comparing endosonography reports with histopathology we have found that the specificity – the potential for endosonography to assess non-involved nodes – is 77%. The sensitivity – the ability to predict lymph node metastasis – is 68%. Accuracy – the ability of endosonography to predict involved and non-involved nodes – is 73%.

This is well short of the accuracy for tumour invasion and an important area of weakness for the technique. No particular histological differences in nodal architecture have so far been found to account for this. With these reservations in mind we have drawn up the following recommendation:

1. Normal lymph nodes are not usually visualised. When no lymph nodes are seen in a patient with rectal cancer the probability of lymph node metastases will be very low.

2. Hyperechoic lymph nodes are not metastatic nodes, but are usually due to non-specific inflammation.
3. Hypoechoic nodes are highly suggestive for lymph node metastases, but inflammatory changes are still possible.

Similar difficulties in interpretation have been found in lymph nodes in the upper gastrointestinal tract (Aibe 1984a; Tio and Tytgat 1984). Endosonography can readily detect lymph node enlargement but precise differentiation between involved and non-involved nodes may be very difficult. None the less endosonography is more accurate than computed tomography (CT).

Palliative Treatment of Rectal Cancer

Some bulky rectal carcinomas in elderly patients are best treated palliatively by laser therapy, transanal resection with a resectoscope or cryosurgery. The aims are to control bleeding, relieve obstruction and avoid a stoma. Endosonography can be used to assess the tumour for depth of penetration to avoid perforation and to assess residual tumour for further treatment.

Impact of Endosonography on Rectal Cancer Management

Although rectal endosonography is not yet widely used it is clear that it may have considerable potential in rectal cancer management. Digital rectal examination is less accurate than endosonography at predicting local invasion and lymph node involvement, and CT scanning is less sensitive for small tumours and early lymph node involvement. Assuming an experienced rectal endosonographer has carried out the examination, and that the scan is correct for depth of invasion and lymph node involvement, how might endosonography help management?

Group 1: Tumour Stage uT1 N0

These are tumours confined to the submucosa, where lymph node involvement has been excluded by endosonography. Taken with other favourable characteristics, such as site, size, numbers of quadrants involved and degree of differentiation, these patients can be treated by local excision. Understaging is unusual in these tumours, but they must still be submitted for careful histological assessment. However, since these comprise only around 10% of rectal cancers, it takes some time to accumulate any experience with these lesions.

Group 2: Tumour Stage uT2 N0

Here the tumour has extended into the muscularis propria, when the risk of lymph node involvement is 10% to 20%. Some of these involved nodes will be detected by endosonography. In younger patients, a conventional radical resection would be indicated, but in selected elderly patients without nodal involvement a local excision could be sensibly employed.

Group 3: Tumour Stage uT2 N1 and uT3 N0

The usual anterior resection or abdominoperineal excision procedures are used for these tumours, but accurate endosonographic staging would allow preoperative selection of patients for adjuvant radiotherapy or chemotherapy.

Group 4: Tumour Stages uT3 N1

This group has a poor prognosis, but still has the potential for cure using adjuvant pre-operative radiotherapy. By identifying involved nodes, selection for radiotherapy could be more accurate and its effect in this particular group assessed.

Group 5: Tumour Stages uT4 N0 and uT4 N1

These are usually bulk cancers which may feel fixed on clinical examination. Fixity is not always due to direct tumour invasion, and endosonography may be able to identify those uT3 tumours fixed by inflammatory tissue. A precise knowledge of the extent and location of local invasion into adjacent pelvic organs will clearly identify patients suitable for pre-operative radiotherapy and indicate those areas where special care would have to be taken during surgery to include involvement "en bloc" with the resection specimen.

UICC Staging of Rectal Cancer

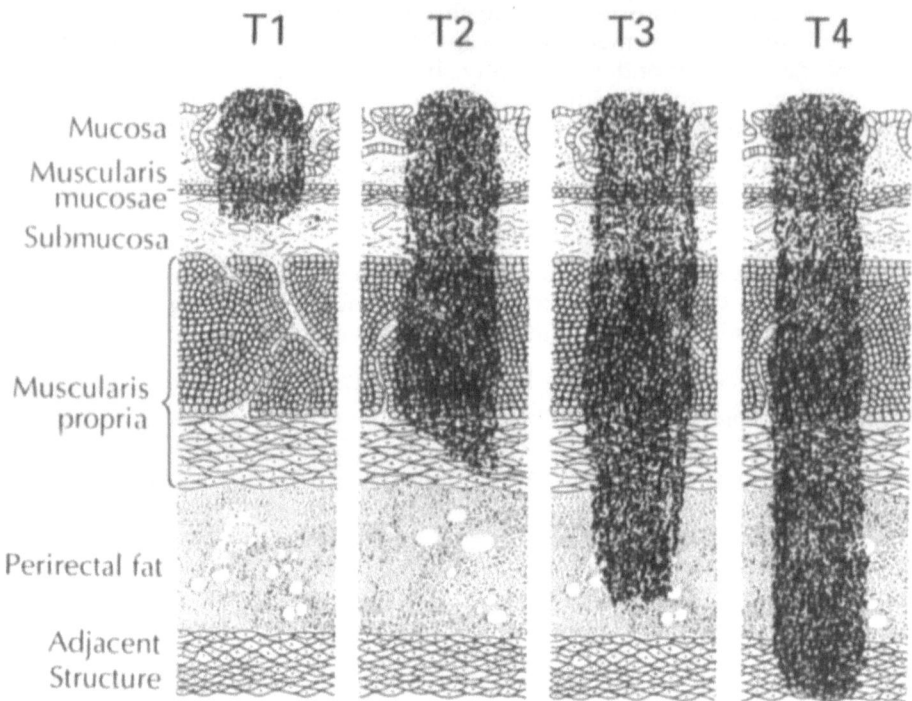

Fig. 6.1. The IUCC TNM staging of local invasion in rectal cancer. Invasion is divided into four stages T1 to T4. (See Appendix.)

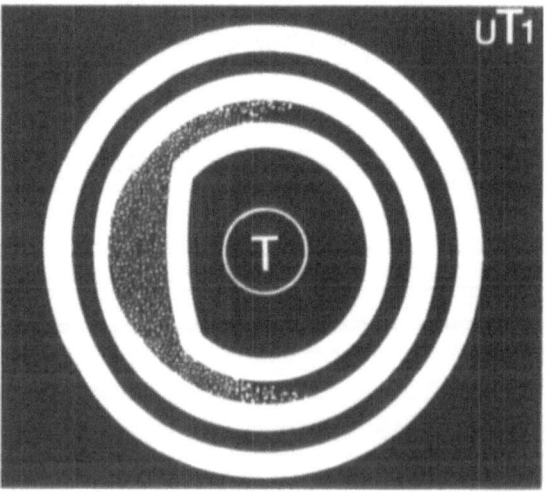

Fig. 6.2. Schematic illustration of the ultrasonic tumour stage uT1. The middle interface representing the borderline between submucosa and muscularis propria is not interrupted. *T*, transducer. (From Feifel et al. 1990, with permission.)

uT1/pT1

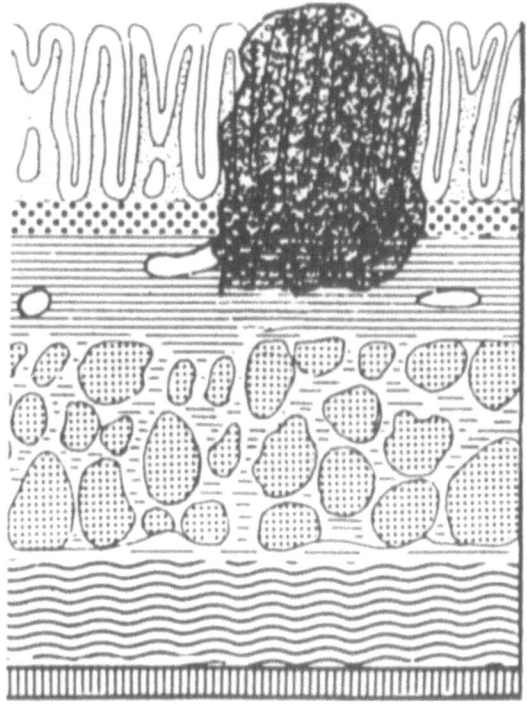

Fig. 6.3. Schematic illustration of the ultrasonic (u) tumour stage $uT1$, which corresponds to the pathohistological (p) stage $pT1$. The tumour does not penetrate muscularis propria. (From Feifel et al. 1990, with permission.)

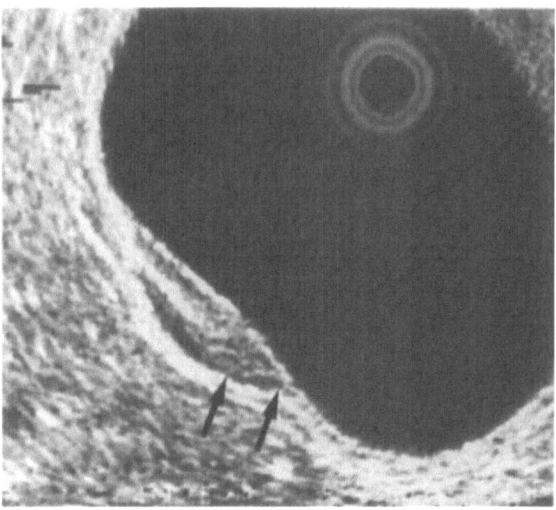

Fig. 6.4. An endosonogram of a small polypoid carcinoma of the rectum (uT1). The tumour is at 7 o'clock and the invasion is limited by the middle layer of submucosa (*arrows*).

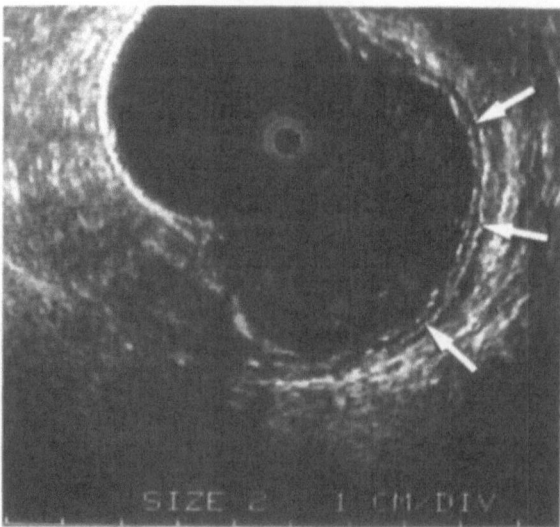

Fig. 6.5. This sonogram is of a large villous carcinoma of the rectum (uT1). The invasion is again limited by the submucosal layer (*arrows*).

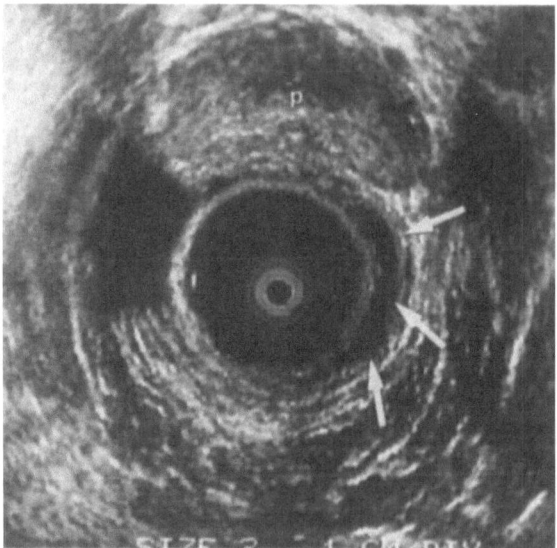

Fig. 6.6. A small uT1 tumour of the rectal wall lying on the right side of the scan (the left side of the patient). The submucosa (*arrowed*) runs around the outside of the lesion. The prostate (*p*) is seen anteriorly.

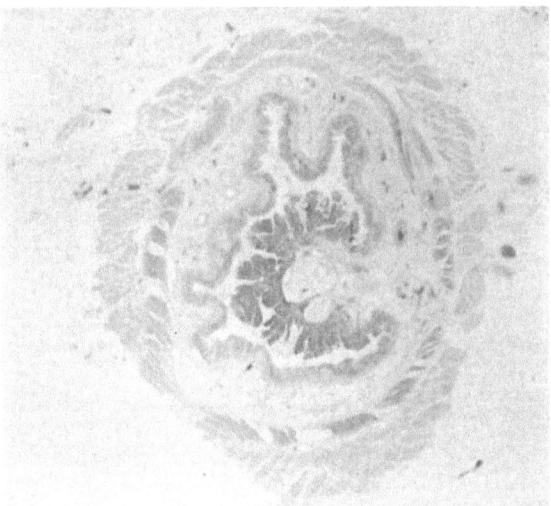

Fig. 6.7. The histological section from the rectum scanned in Fig. 6.6. A polypoid carcinoma of the rectal wall is present and the submucosa is intact.

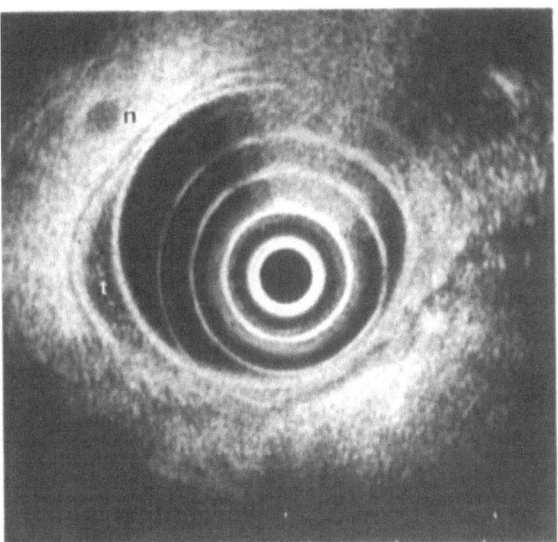

Fig. 6.8. With 12 MHz transducer (Olympus). T1 tumour (*t*) with hyperechoic lymph node (*n*) at top right.

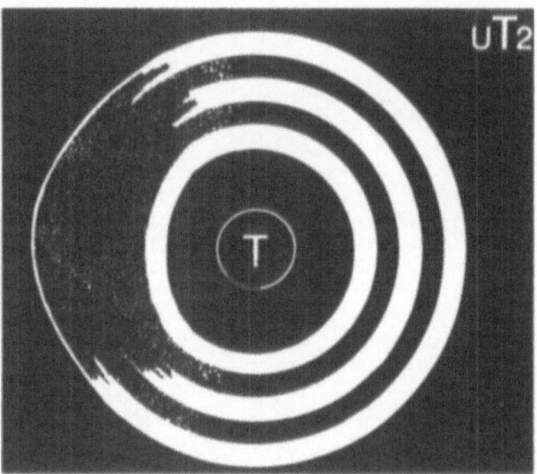

Fig. 6.9. Schematic illustration of the sonographic tumour stage uT2. The middle interface is interrupted whereas the outer interface, representing the borderline with the perirectal fat, is intact. T, transducer. (From Feifel et al. 1990, with permission.)

uT2/pT2

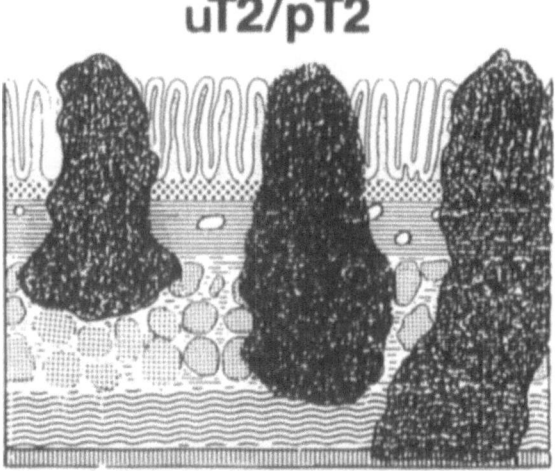

Fig. 6.10. Schematic illustration of tumour stage uT2 corresponding to pT2. Tumour does not penetrate through the muscularis propria or serosa. (From Feifel et al. 1990, with permission.)

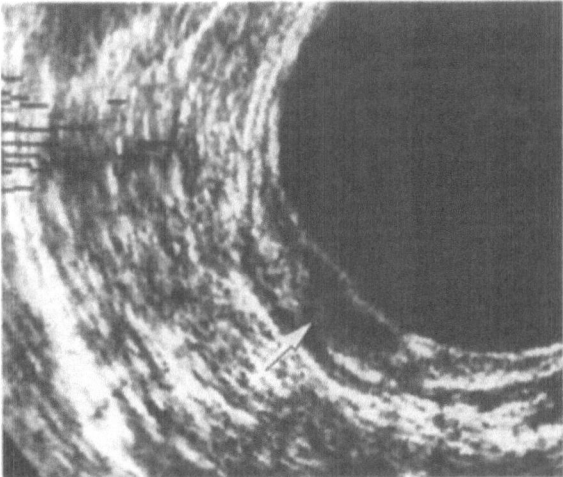

Fig. 6.11. An endosonogram of a uT2 tumour. The small carcinoma (*arrowed*) on this occasion has eroded through the submucosa into the muscularis propria. Containment by the muscularis propria is evident from the good interface between it and the surrounding fat.

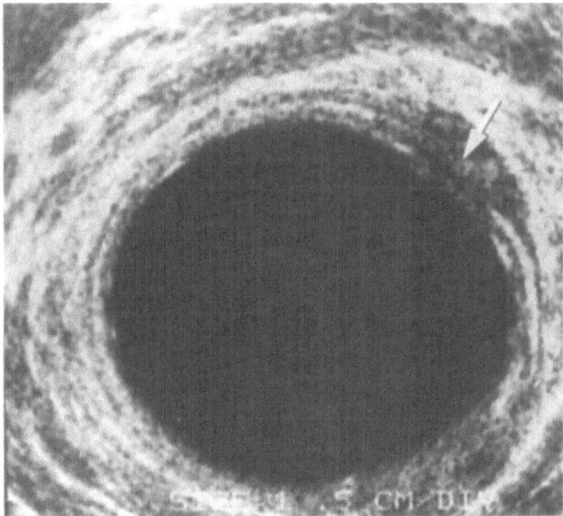

Fig. 6.12. A small uT2 tumour of the rectum (*arrowed*). The submucosal middle layer has been destroyed indicating invasion into the muscularis propria.

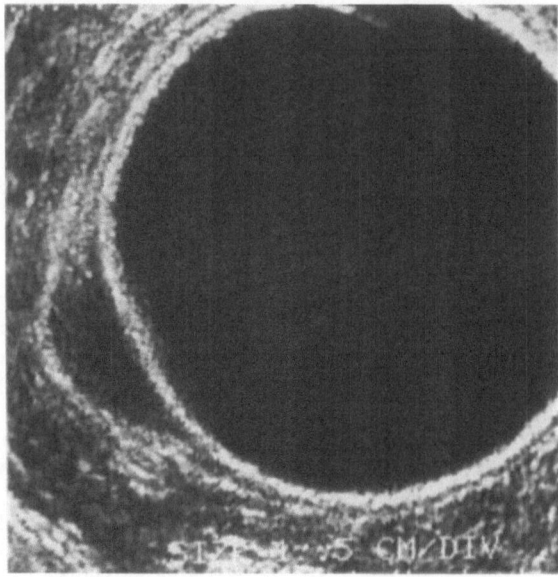

Fig. 6.13. Tumour uT2. Middle hyperechoic layer has disappeared indicating tumour invasion into the muscularis propria.

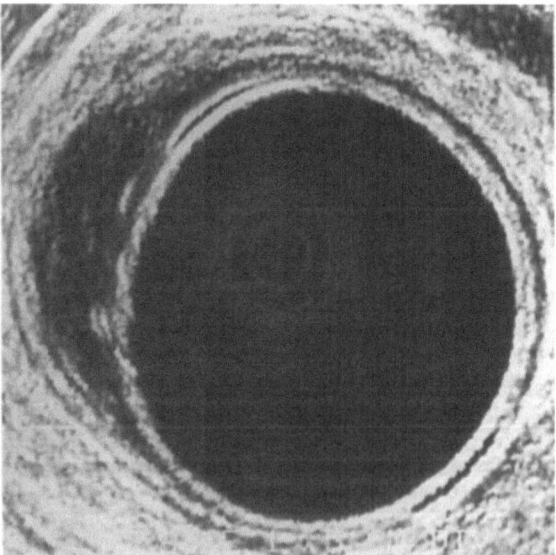

Fig. 6.14. Tumour uT2. Again the middle hyperechoic layer has been disrupted.

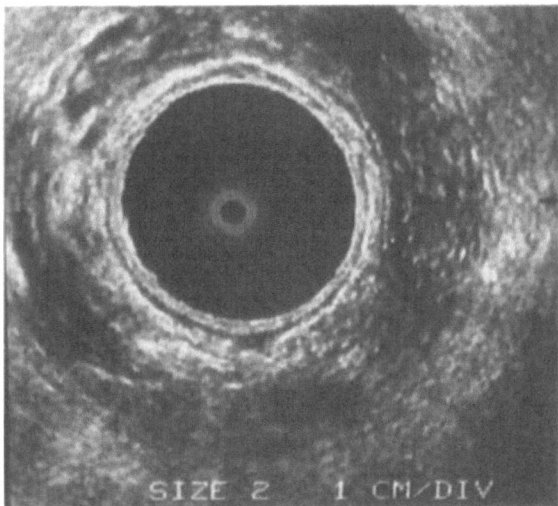

Fig. 6.15. There are various degress of invasion displayed here and in Figs. 6.16 and 6.17, taken from the examination of one patient. The patient examined had an ulcerating lesion which at this point in the rectum is not visible. A five-layered normal rectal wall is seen.

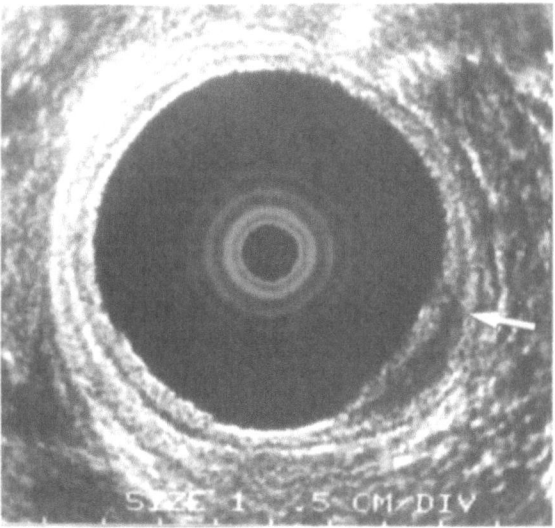

Fig. 6.16. In contrast slightly higher in the rectum there is now a lesion which is limited by the submucosal layer (*arrows*).

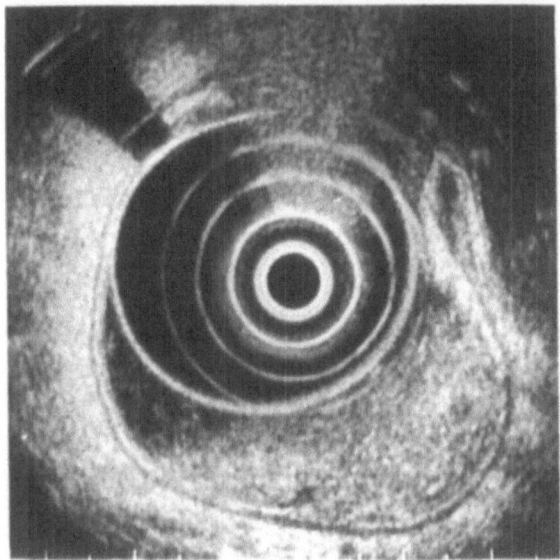

Fig. 6.17. With 12 MHz transducer (Olympus). T2 tumour, minimal infiltration of the muscularis seen at histology.

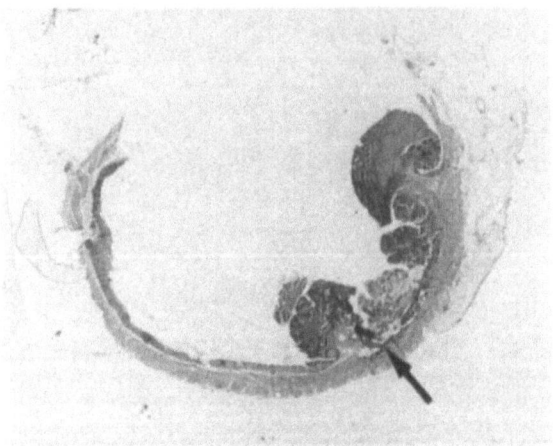

Fig. 6.18. This histological section from the resected specimen of Fig. 6.17 shows that the ultrasonic prediction of extent of local invasion was correct with the ulcerating tumour just invading the muscularis propria (*arrow*).

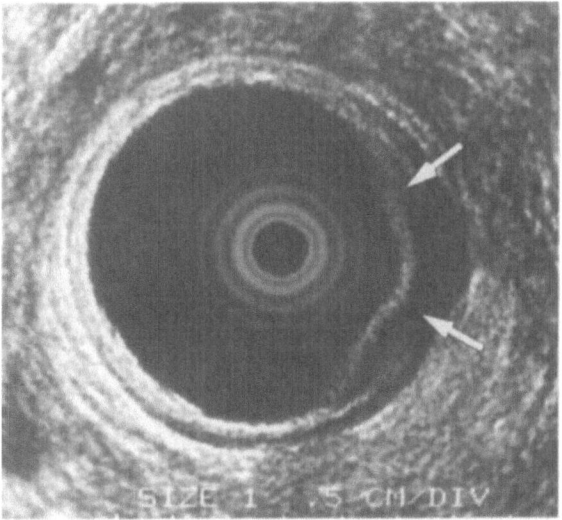

Fig. 6.19. This uT2 tumour has now invaded through the submucosa into the muscularis propria (*arrows*) but has not progressed any further.

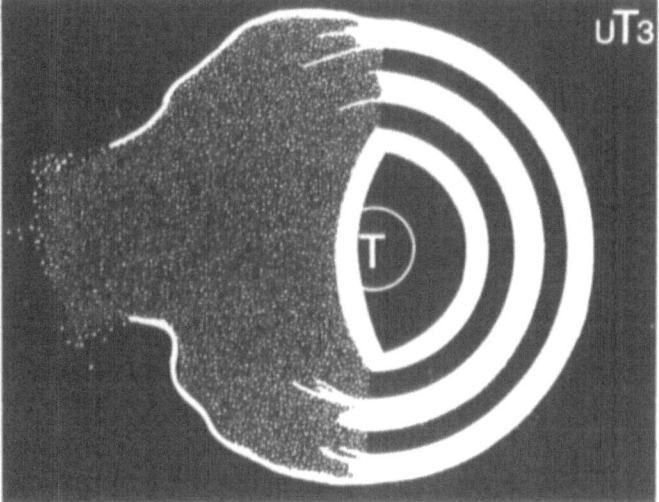

Fig. 6.20. Schematic illustration of the sonographic tumour stage uT3. The outer interface has been disrupted by the penetrating tumour. *T*, transducer. (From Feifel et al. 1990, with permission.)

uT3/pT3

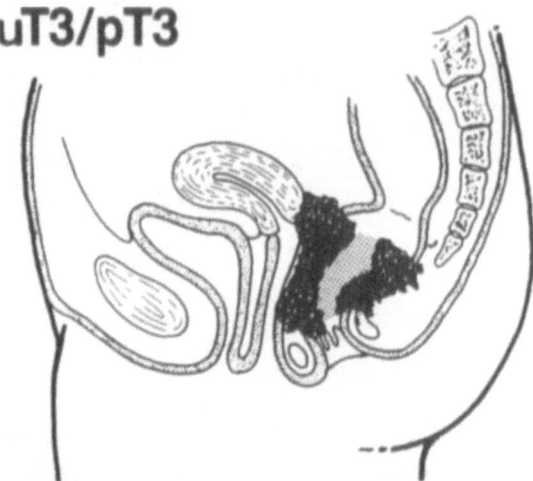

Fig. 6.21. Schematic illustration of tumour stage uT3 corresponding to pT3. Tumour penetrates into the perirectal area or into neighbouring organs. (From Feifel et al. 1990, with permission.)

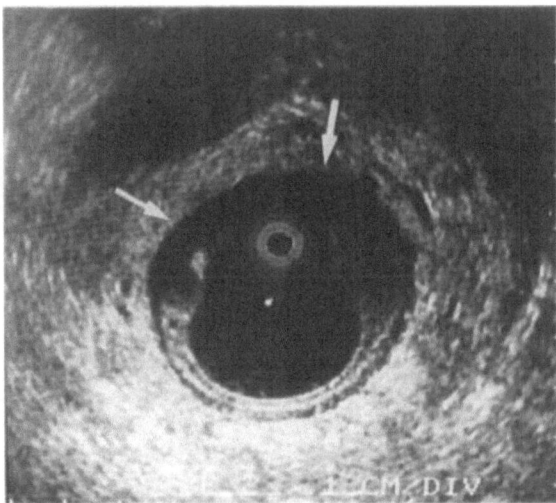

Fig. 6.22. In this example of a uT3 tumour of the anterior rectal wall there is invasion through all the ultrasonic layers indicating spread into the mesorectal fat (*arrows*).

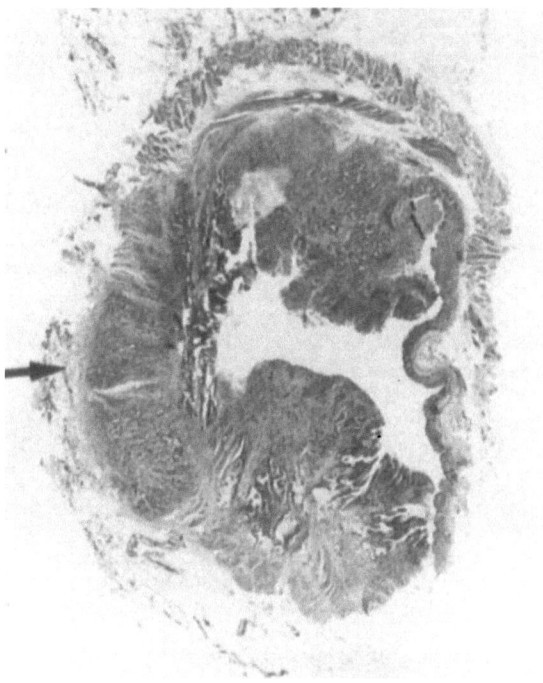

Fig. 6.23. This is a transverse histological section of the tumour scanned in Fig. 6.22. On the left side of the section it is apparent that the tumour has invaded out into the mesorectal fat (*arrow*).

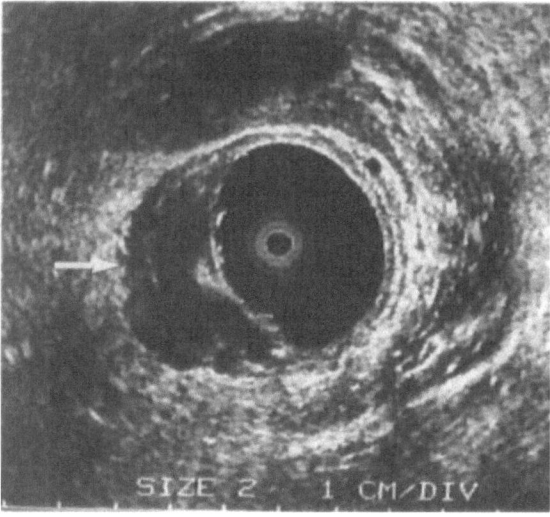

Fig. 6.24. A uT3 tumour. The outer border is irregular, indicating invasion of the mesorectum (*arrow*).

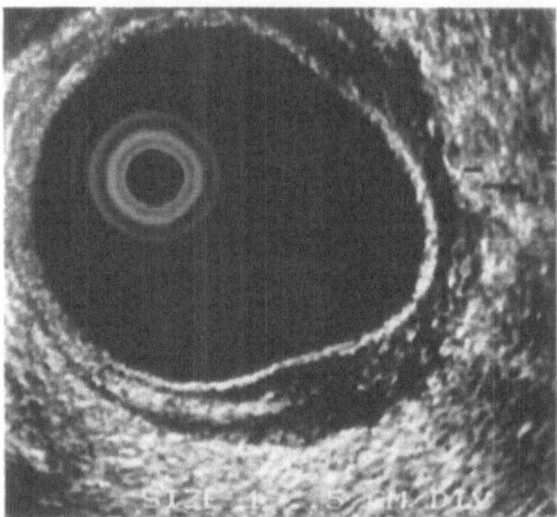

Fig. 6.25. A uT3 tumour.

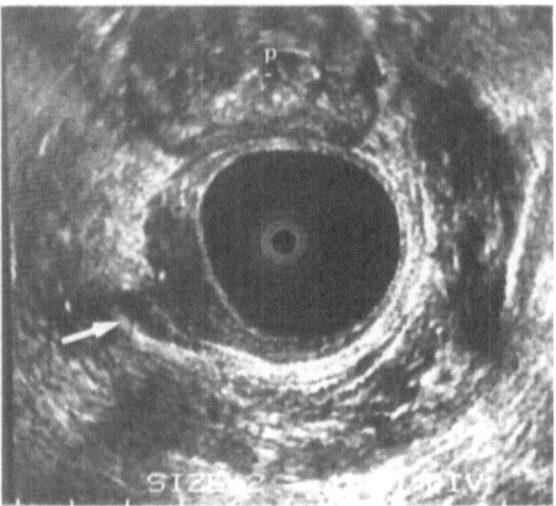

Fig. 6.26. This male patient had a tumour of the lower rectum at the level of the prostate (*p*) which can be seen anteriorly in this scan. The tumour on the left-hand side of the scan invades through all layers (*arrow*).

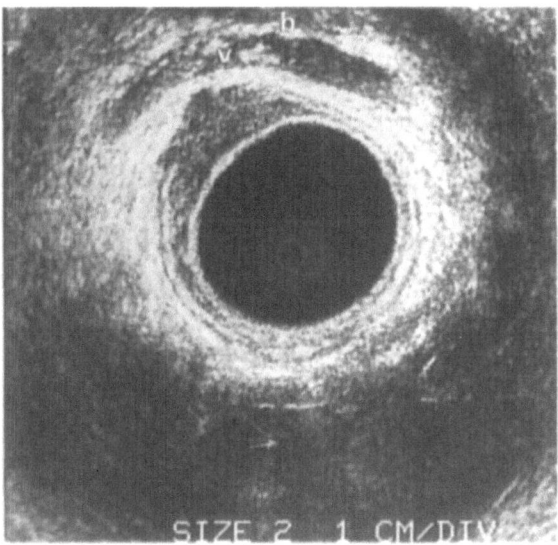

Fig. 6.27. A uT3 tumour with slight penetration into perirectal fat. Female patient. *b*, bladder; *v*, vagina.

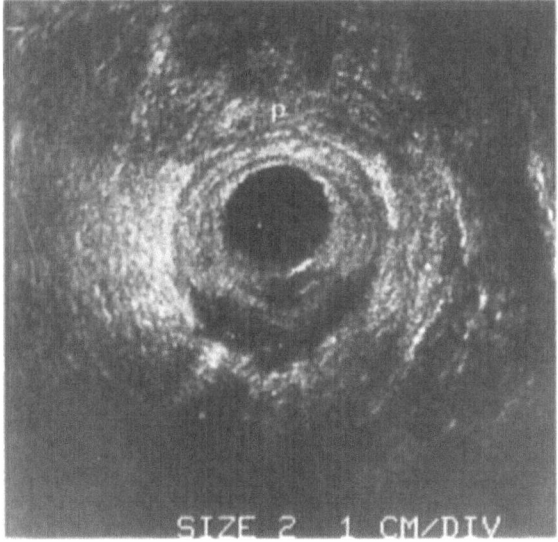

Fig. 6.28 A uT3 tumour near the anal canal (anorectal junction) producing thickening of the rectal wall. The prostate is also visible anteriorly (*p*).

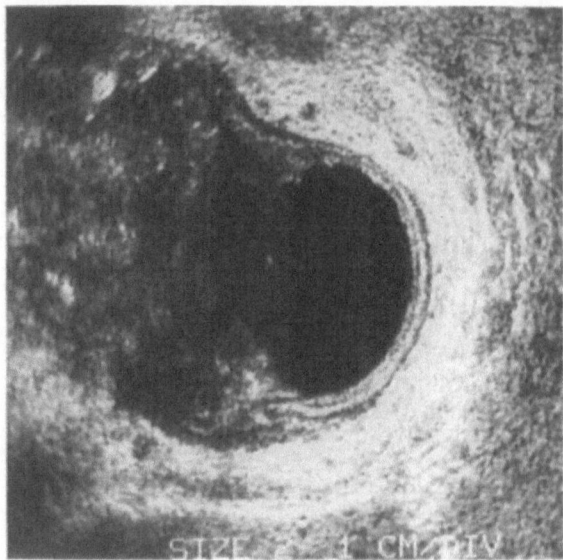

Fig. 6.29. A uT3 tumour with massive local extension.

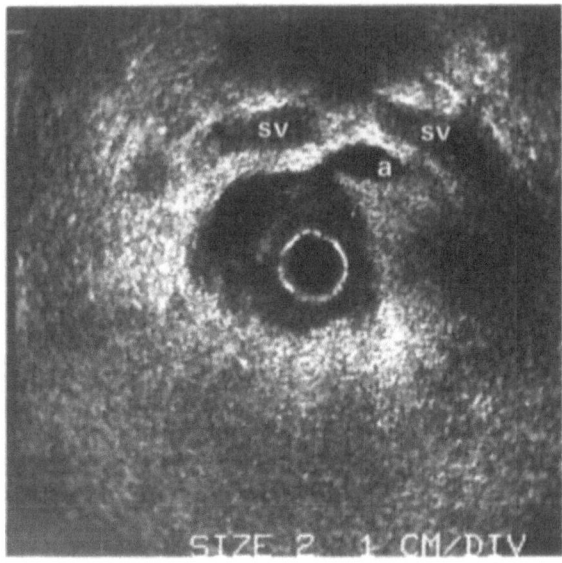

Fig. 6.30. Circular rectal cancer with stenosis of the lumen and perforation into perirectal fat. The abscess area is hypoechoic with no structures. There is no definite invasion of local structures; therefore the tumour is stage uT3. *sv*, seminal vesicles; *a*, abscess.

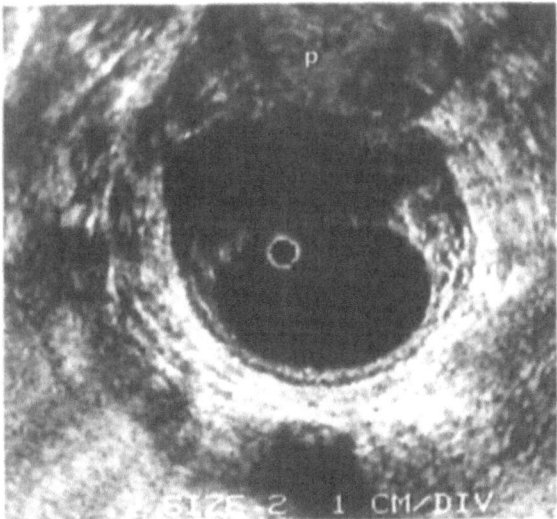

Fig. 6.31. uT4 tumour invading anteriorly into the prostate gland (*p*).

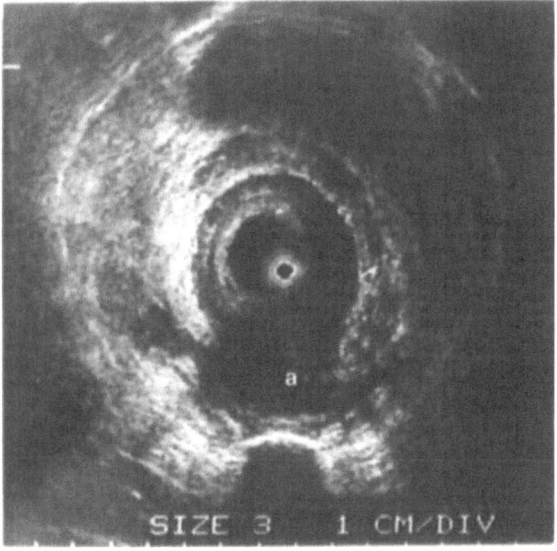

Fig. 6.32. In this example of a uT4 tumour there is a hypoechoic area behind the rectum which is a retrorectal abscess (*a*). At a higher level the tumour had eroded the sacrum.

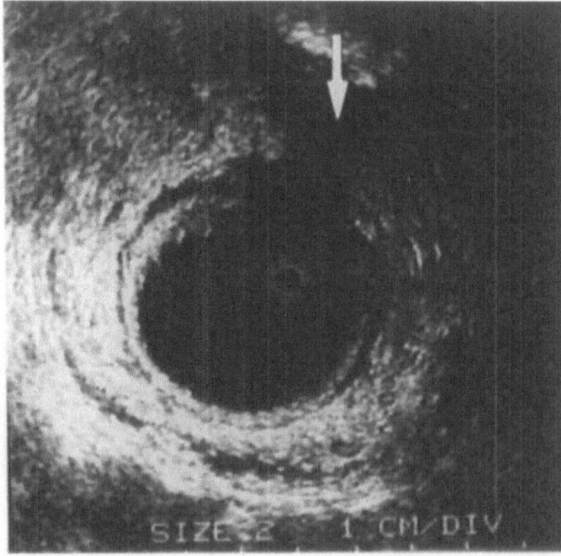

Fig. 6.33. The same uT4 tumour at a higher level. Here the tumour is invading the bladder (*arrow*).

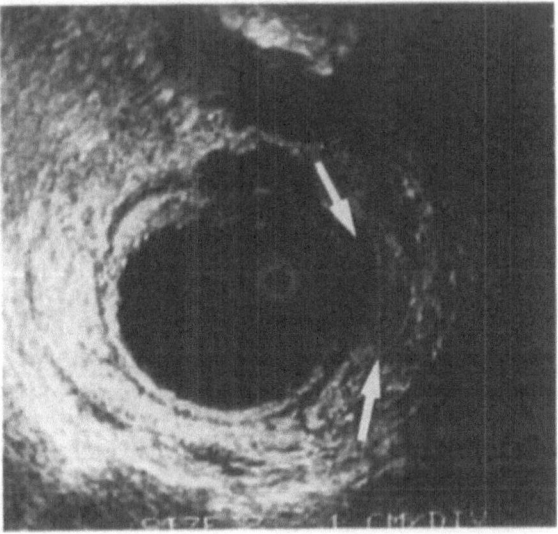

Fig. 6.34. A uT4 tumour. At this level the local extension is nearing the bladder anteriorly (*arrow*).

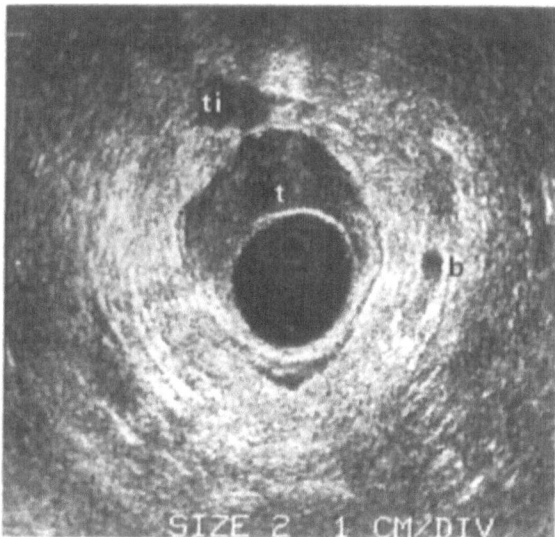

Fig. 6.35. A uT4 tumour at the anterior rectal wall, with an area which seems to be free tumour metastasis but which the sonogram of only a few millimetres upwards shows to be tumour spread in continuity. *t*, tumour; *ti*, tumour island; *b*, blood vessel.

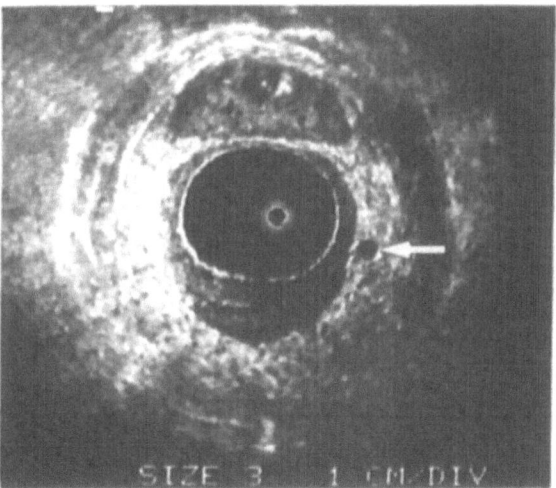

Fig. 6.36. This patient with a uT3 rectal tumour had one small nodal metastasis (*arrowed*).

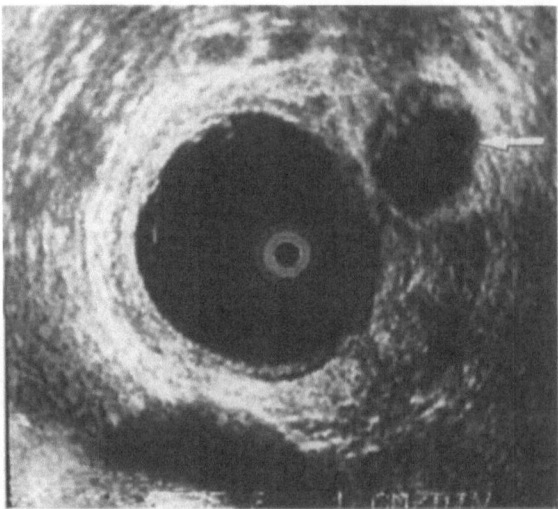

Fig. 6.37. At a different level in the same patient a large area with similar ultrasonic characteristics was imaged (*arrow*). Histopathologically, this contained tumour but no lymphoid tissue.

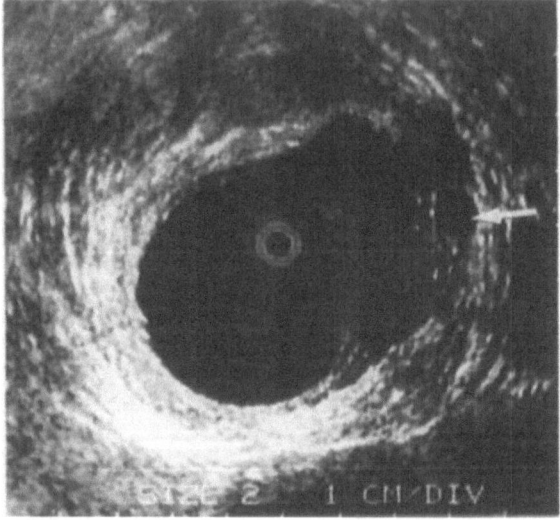

Fig. 6.38. Nodal metastases cannot be distinguished ultrasonically from islands of extramural tumour. This and the next scan illustrate this point. Here there is a quite definite hypechoic area (*arrowed*), which was correctly predicted as a nodal metastasis.

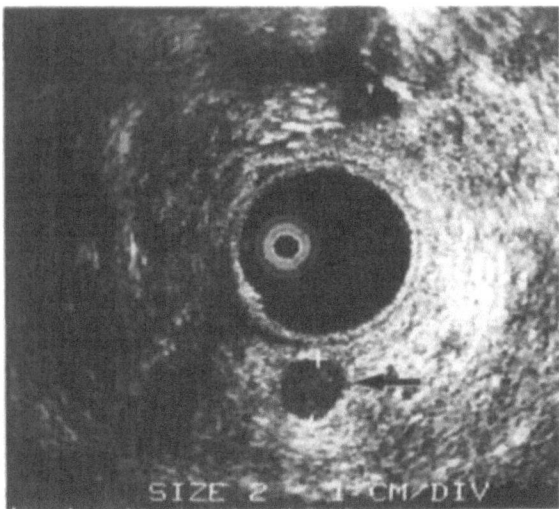

Fig. 6.39. Slightly higher in the rectum a larger nodal metastasis was also identified (*arrow*). This measured just over 1 cm in diameter.

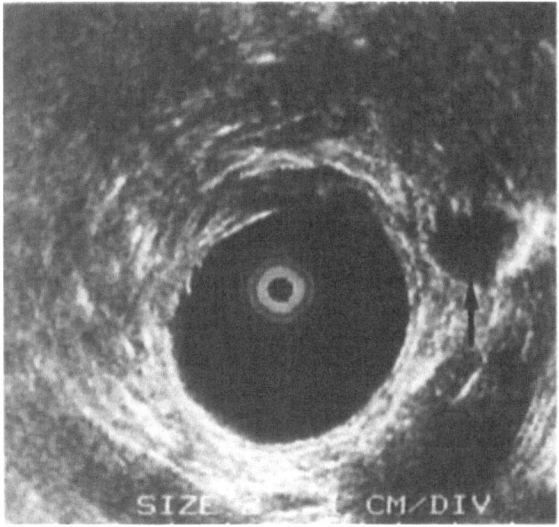

Fig. 6.40. This scan also shows a hypoechoic area outside the rectal wall at the 2 o'clock position (*arrow*). On histopathological examination, there were a number of small involved nodes matted together.

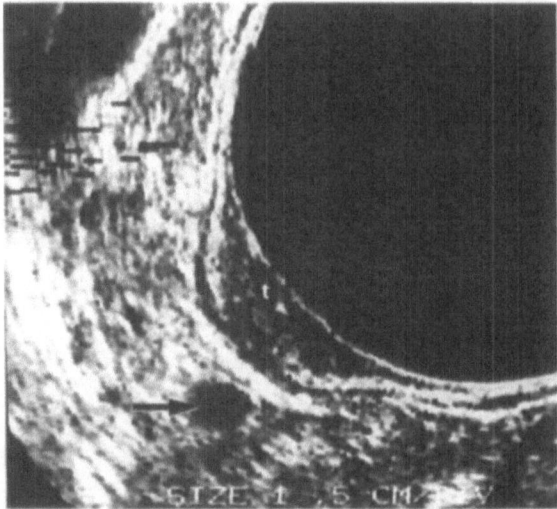

Fig. 6.41. This is an example of a false positive node (*arrow*) in a patient with a uT2 tumour (*t*).

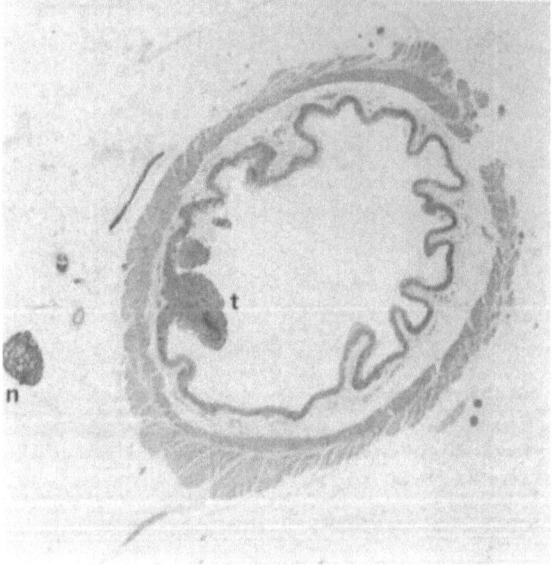

Fig. 6.42. This is the histopathological section from the scan shown in Fig. 6.41. The node (*n*) has been accurately identified but microscopically contained no tumour (*t*).

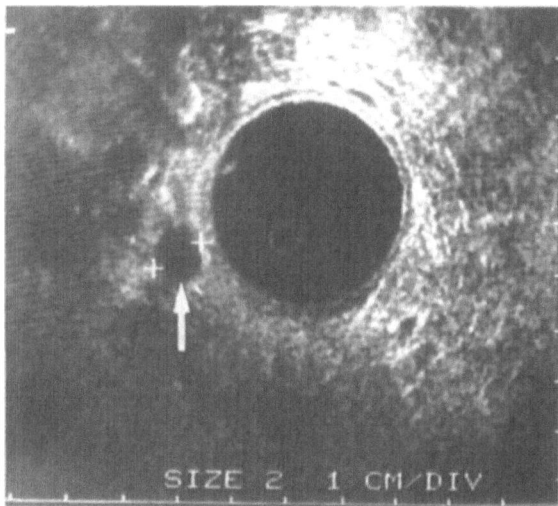

Fig. 6.43. Blood vessels in cross-section may be mistaken for lymph nodes. An example of this is shown here (*arrow*), with the vessel having a circumscribed hypoechoic appearance.

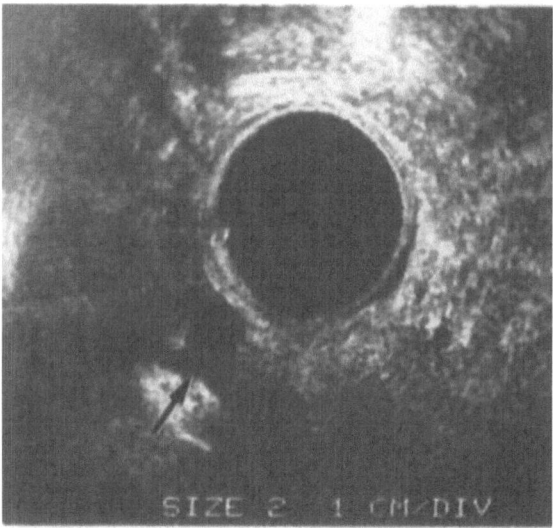

Fig. 6.44. By moving the endoprobe, however, the vessels seen in the previous image can be demonstrated to branch, which distinguishes them from nodes (*arrow*).

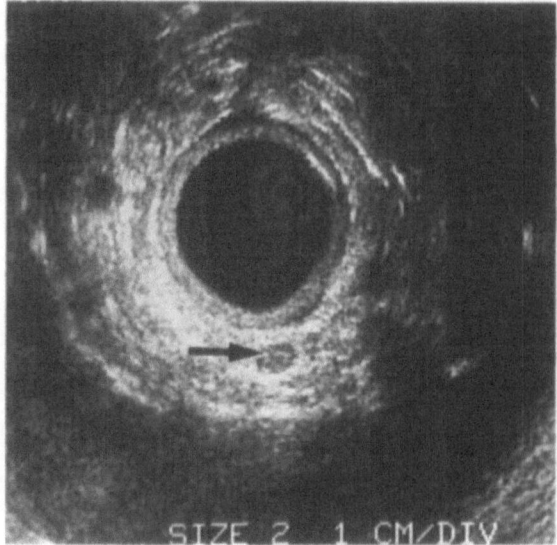

Fig. 6.45. Hyperechoic lymph node (*arrow*).

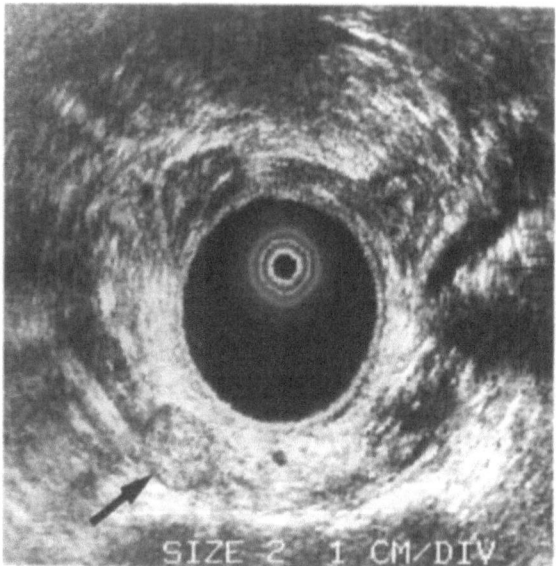

Fig. 6.46. Hyperechoic lymph node (*arrow*).

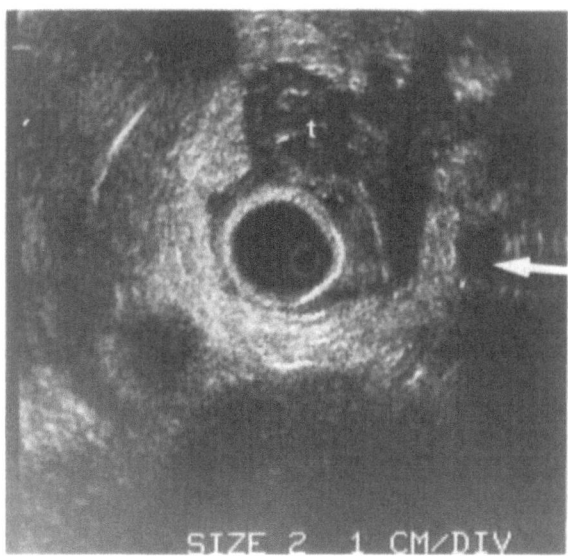

Fig. 6.47. A uT3 tumour (*t*) with hypoechoic lymph node (*arrow*).

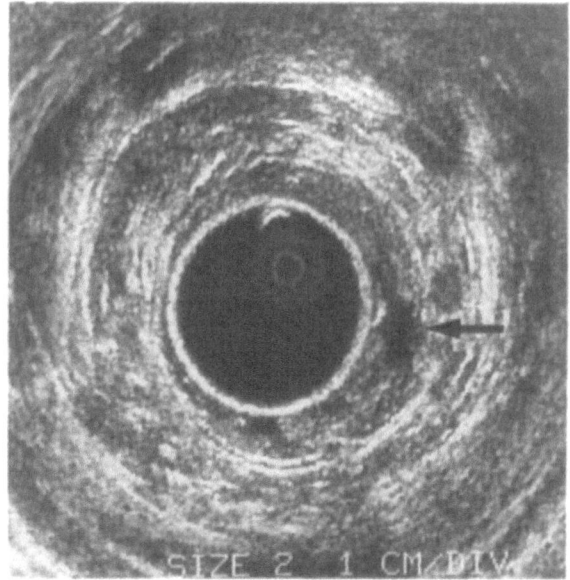

Fig. 6.48. Hyperechoic node (*arrow*).

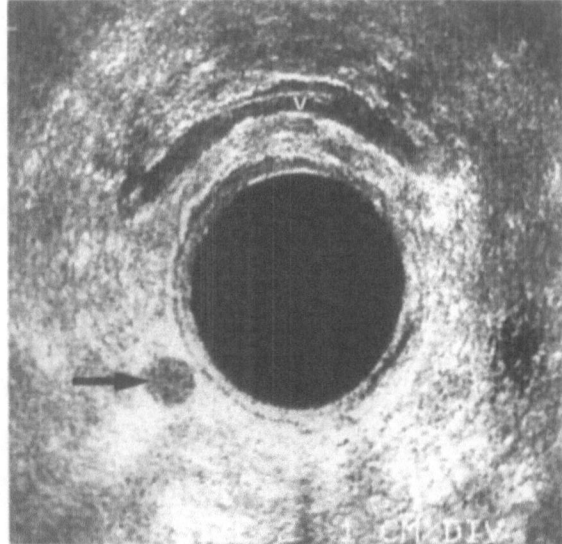

Fig. 6.49. Hyperechoic node (*arrow*). *v*, vagina.

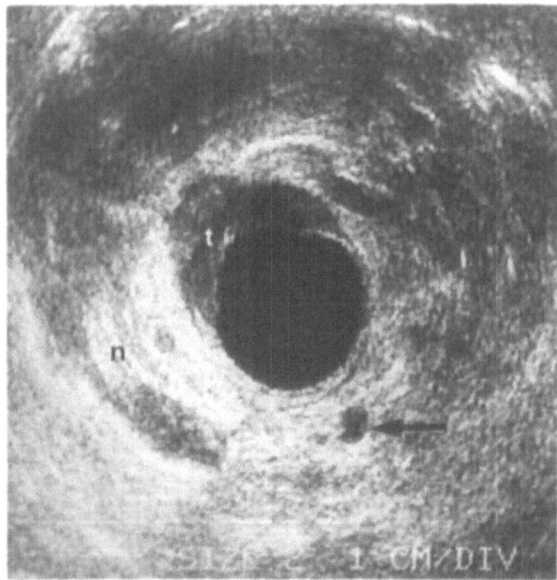

Fig. 6.50. A uT3 tumour (*t*), with hypoechoic (*arrow*) and hyperechoic nodes (*n*).

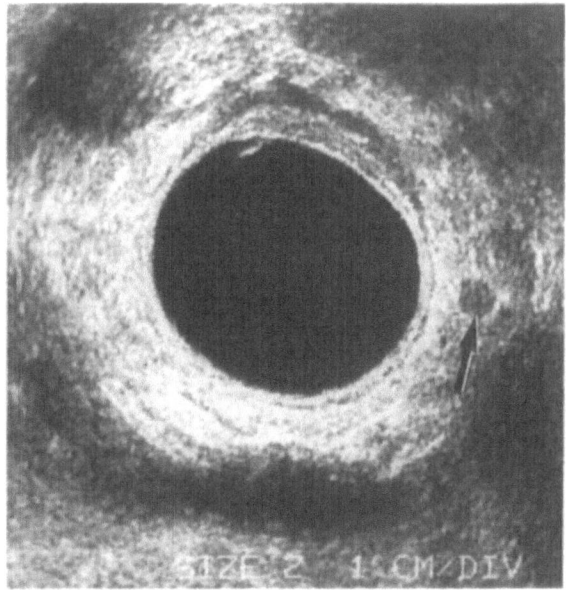

Fig. 6.51. A T3 tumour and hyperechoic node (*arrow*).

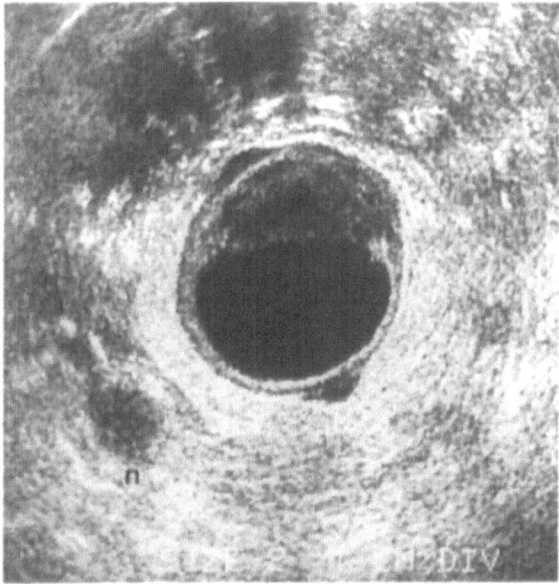

Fig. 6.52. Hypoechoic lymph node (*n*) 1.5 cm in diameter.

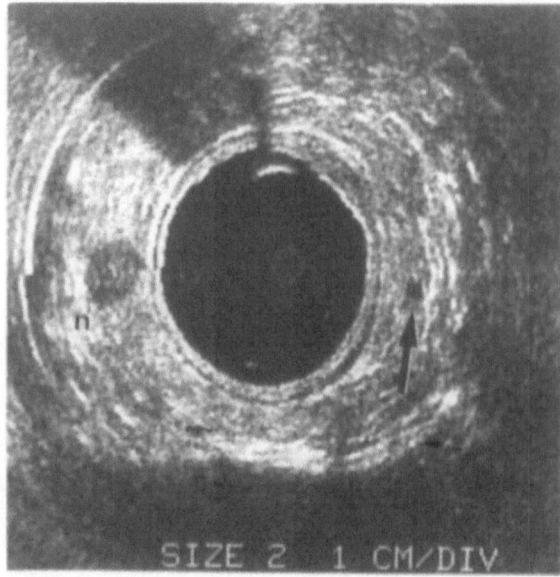

Fig. 6.53. Hyperechoic lymph node (*n*) 1.2 cm in diameter. There is a blood vessel at right (*arrow*).

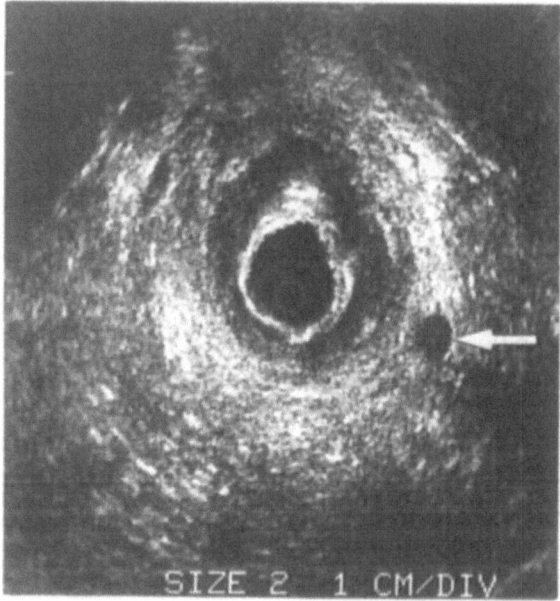

Fig. 6.54. Hypoechoic node (*arrow*) beside the upper part of the anal canal.

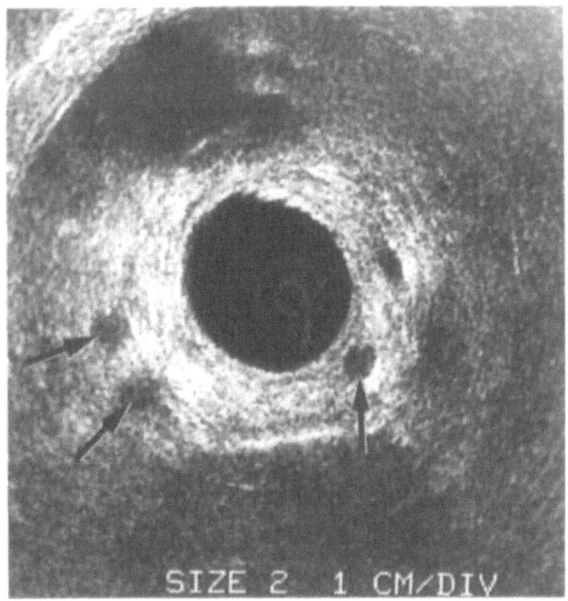

Fig. 6.55. Hypoechoic nodes (*arrows*).

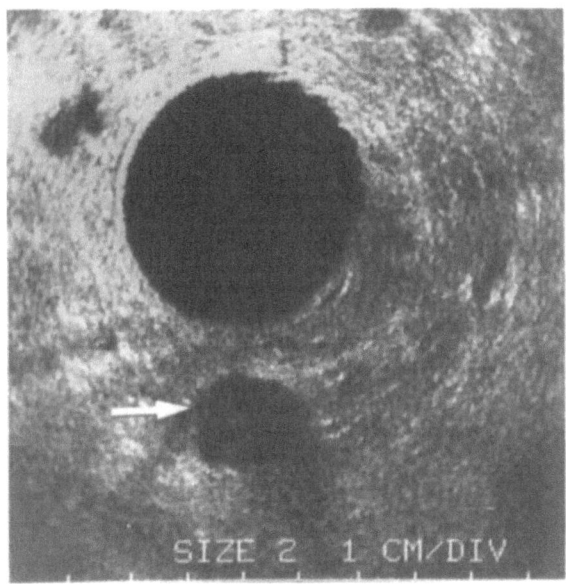

Fig. 6.56. Hypoechoic node 2.0 cm in diameter (*arrow*).

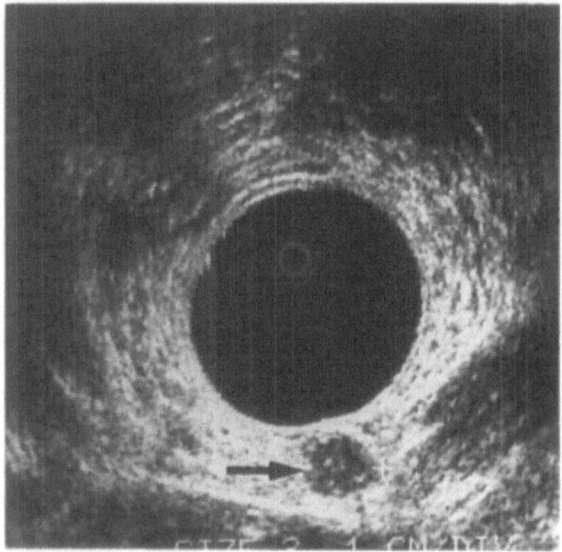

Fig. 6.57. Lymph node (*arrow*) seen by ultrasound 6 months after local excision of a pT2 rectal cancer. Second-look operation and histology revealed metastasis. (Note mixed echogenicity of the lymph node – neither hypo nor hyper!)

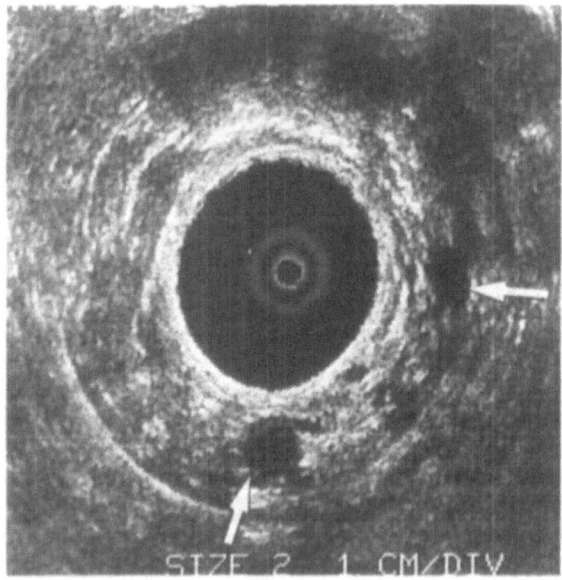

Fig. 6.58. Hypoechoic lymph nodes (*arrows*).

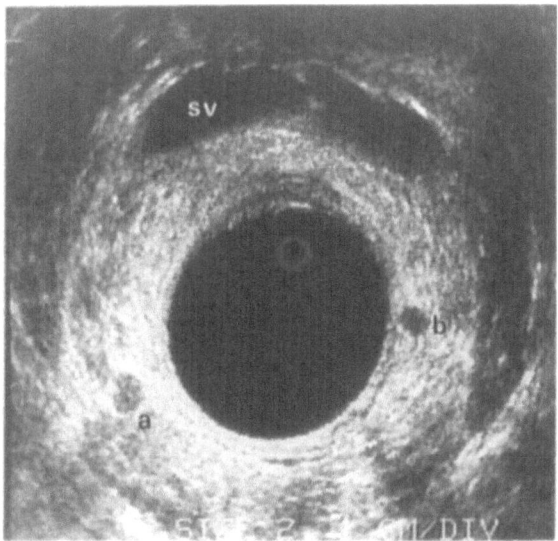

Fig. 6.59. Hyperechoic (*a*) and relatively hypoechoic (*b*) nodes. Both were non-specifically inflamed on histological examination. Seminal vesicles (*sv*) are seen anteriorly.

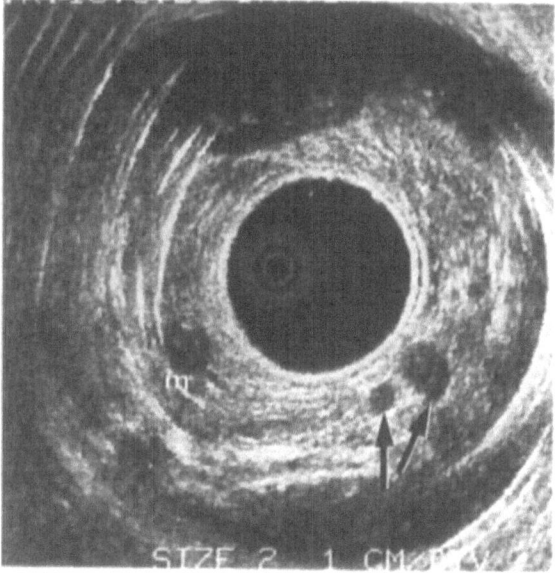

Fig. 6.60. Relatively hyperechoic nodes. On the left a micrometastasis (*m*), on the right two nodes with non-specific inflammation at histology (*arrows*).

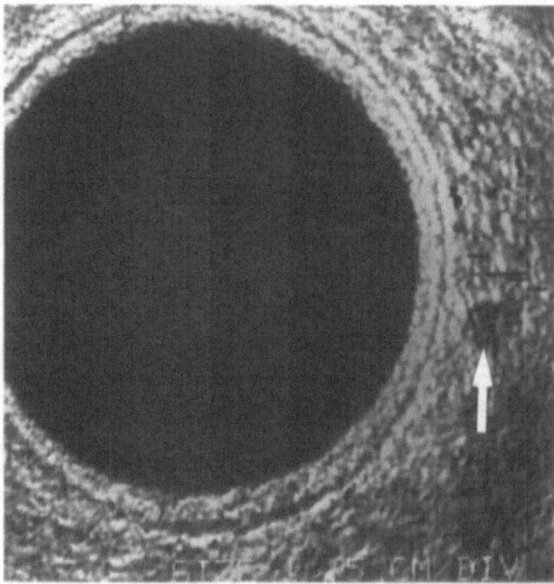

Fig. 6.61. Small lymph node (*arrow*): fat-like echogenicity 3 to 4 mm. This was seen 3 months after local excision of a T2 rectal cancer and disappeared 3 months later.

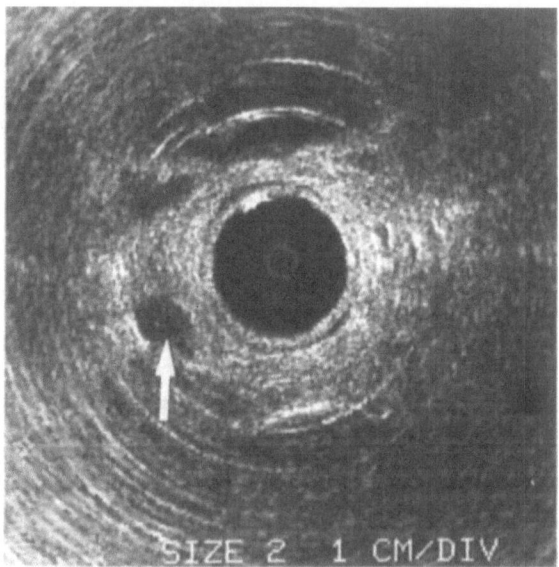

Fig. 6.62. Hypoechoic lymph node metastasis (*arrow*).

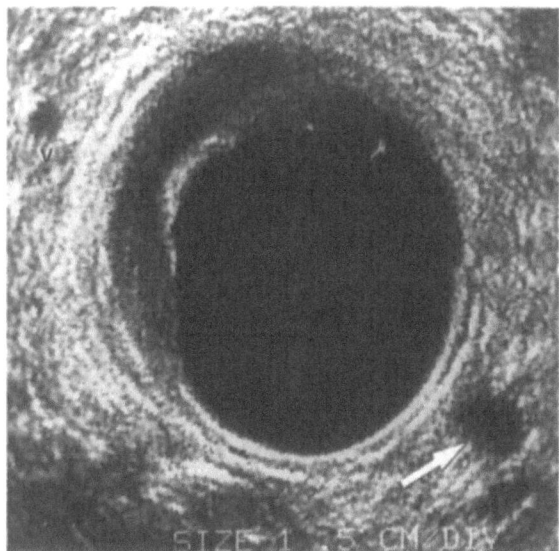

Fig. 6.63. A uT2 tumour with hypoechoic lymph node metastasis (bottom right: *arrow*). Note the blood vessel (upper left: *v*).

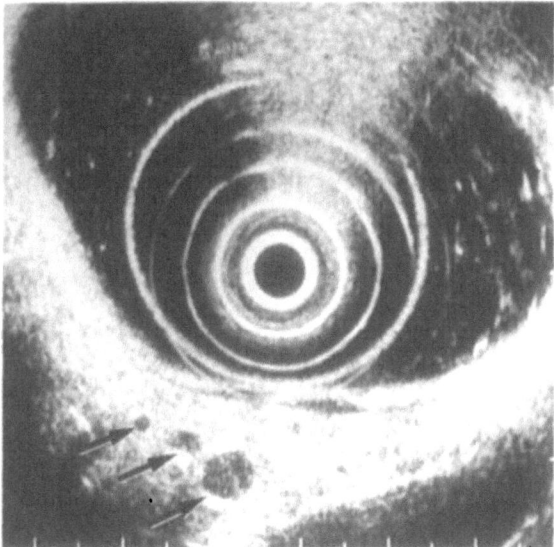

Fig. 6.64. With Olympus 12 MHz transducer. Three hyperechoic lymph nodes in the mesorectum – non-involved and all 5 mm or less in diameter (*arrows*).

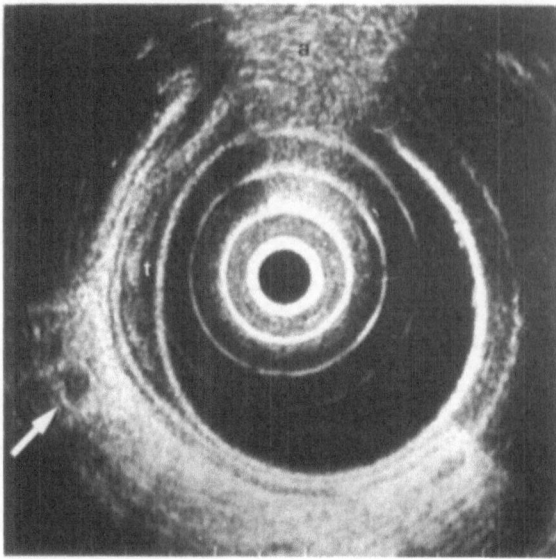

Fig. 6.65. With Olympus 12 MHz transducer. T1 tumour (*t*) on the right with hyperechoic lymph node (*arrow*). The brighter shadow around the node may indicate tumour involvement. There is an artefact (*a*) anteriorly.

7 Local Recurrence

Although there are only a few studies using endosonography at regular intervals following surgery this is potentially a very important application (Figs. 7.1 to 7.18). After a restorative anterior resection of the rectum for rectal cancer the incidence of local recurrence is between 5% and 20%. The peak interval for the development of recurrence is 1 to 2 years following surgery. Local recurrence may occur as a result of an inadequate distal resection margin, inadequate clearance of the mesorectum, inadequate lateral clearance, or tumour implantation of viable lumenal cancer cells at the time of surgery. It may present as a mass outside the rectal wall near the anastomotic site, or as an anastomotic recurrence. True anastomotic recurrence is rare and frequent endoscopy and careful evaluation of a suture line are unlikely to have a major impact on recurrence.

We have used rectal endosonography at 3-monthly intervals after anterior resection in order to try to detect local recurrence at an early stage, and the results are promising.

Preparation

As for any examination good preparation with enemata is essential. The anastomosis will usually be slightly narrower than the surrounding rectum or even stenosed and a rectoscope is first passed through the anastomosis, which is carefully inspected. The ultrasound probe is then placed through the rectoscope so that it is lying above the anastomosis. The rectum is then scanned from above downwards. The anastomosis often grips the balloon or distorts it and the volume of water in the balloon has to be varied considerably to obtain optimal views.

Normal Appearance

Assessment of the pelvis following surgery is more difficult than in the pre-operative case. The anastomotic site is usually narrowed and thickened, and the normal rectal wall echo pattern cannot be discerned. Collections of fluid outside the rectal wall or prolapsing loops of small bowel can be confusing and the distinction between an abscess, recurrence, or a pelvic peritoneal cyst can be a problem. With practice, however, a normal expected range of appearances will become clear. The staples of stapling devices do not interfere with sonographic interpretation (Fig. 7.2). They are usually brightly hyperechoic and cast only a short narrow shadow.

Recurrence

Local recurrence has an appearance similar to that of primary rectal cancer. It is hypoechoic, but not always homogeneous and may have either a sharp or a blurred edge. It does, however, look quite different from the surrounding perirectal fat (Fig. 7.3). Islands of recurrent tumour as small as 5 mm can be detected. The pitfalls to diagnosis are collections of fluid, granulation tissue or loops of small bowel. For these reasons a suspected recurrence on endosonography must be biopsied, or carefully documented and the examination repeated after an interval. In these circumstances if the same changes are again seen or if there is progression and enlargement of the lesion then recurrence is highly likely.

Biopsies can be carried out under anaesthesia transrectally or transperineally, and ultrasound can be used to guide the biopsy needle.

Vaginal Endosonography

Female patients who have had an abdominoperineal excision for carcinoma of the rectum can be scanned per vaginam for local recurrence. The anatomy is more difficult to interpret without the landmark of the rectal wall.

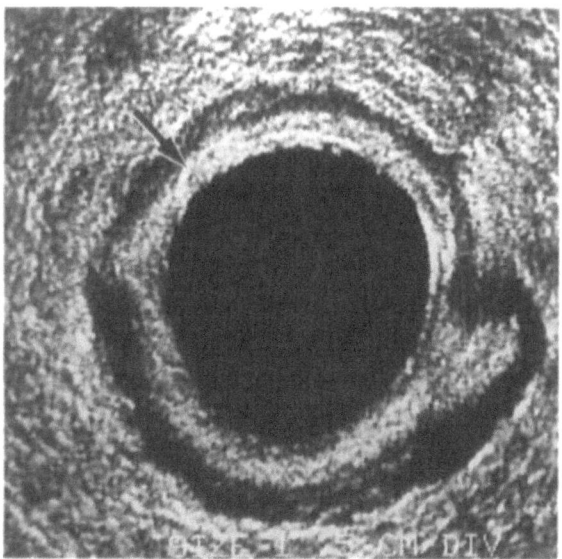

Fig. 7.1. Typical hand-sewn anastomosis. Note the thickened layers (*arrow*).

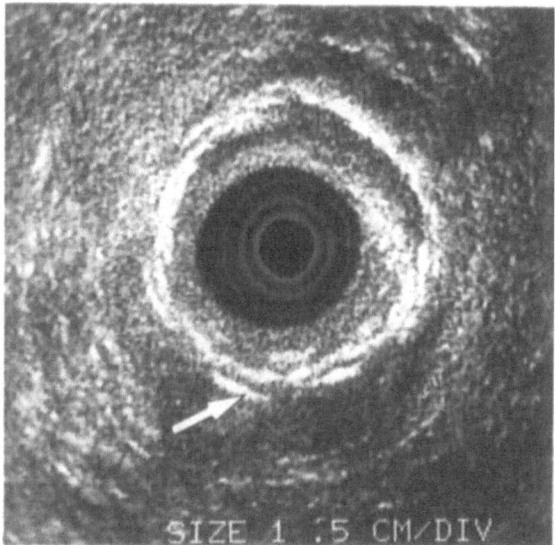

Fig. 7.2. Stapled anastomosis. The staples give hyperechoic reflections (*arrow*) but do not cast shadows or obscure the sonogram.

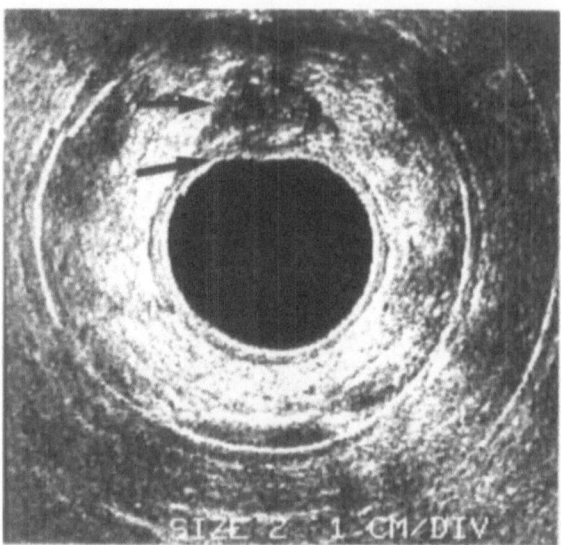

Fig. 7.3. Recurrent rectal cancer anteriorly. Note the intact inner layers (*arrow*) and the hypoechoic appearance of primary rectal cancer.

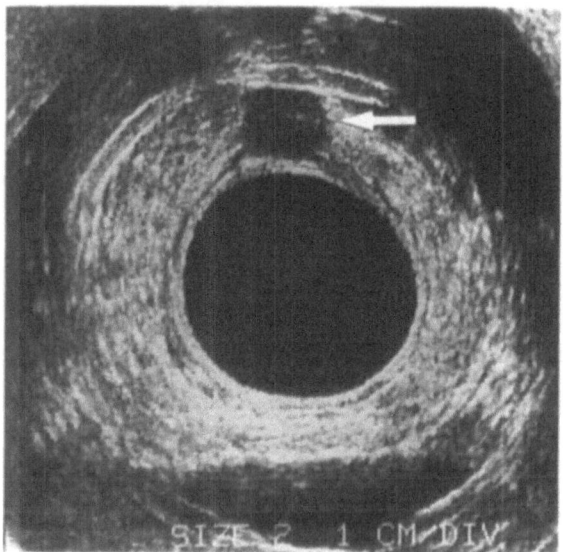

Fig. 7.4. Local recurrence anteriorly (*arrow*).

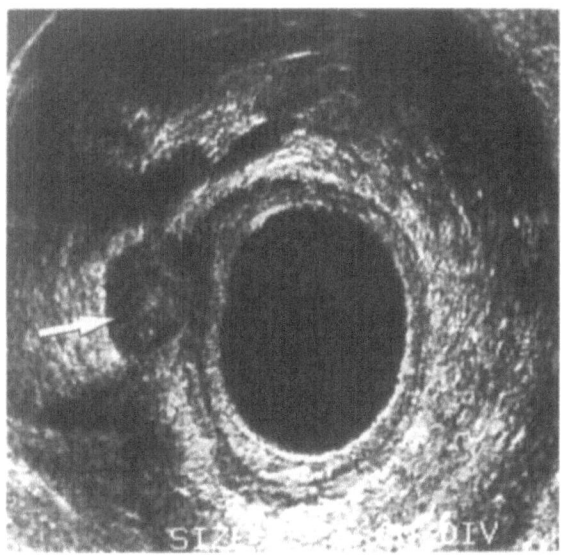

Fig. 7.5. Local recurrence outside the endoscopically intact rectal wall (*arrow*).

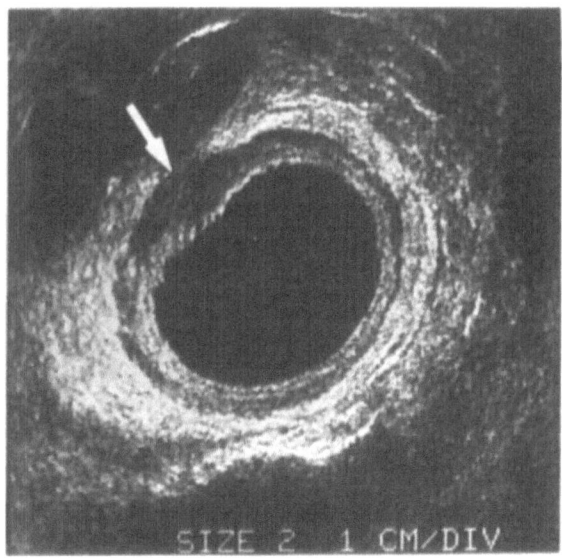

Fig. 7.6. Local recurrence (*arrow*).

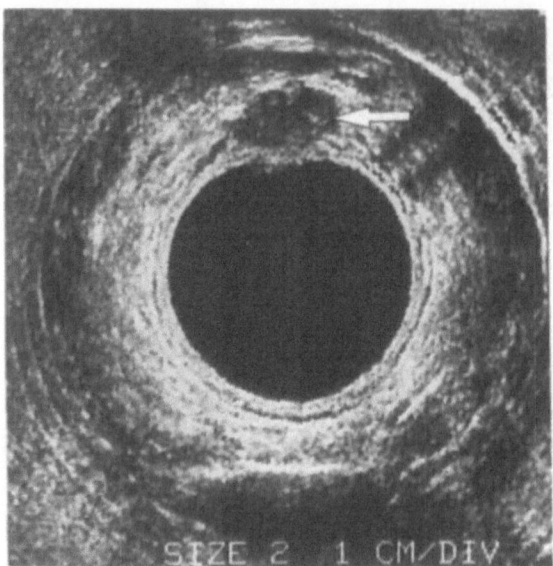

Fig. 7.7. Local recurrence after anterior resection (*arrow*).

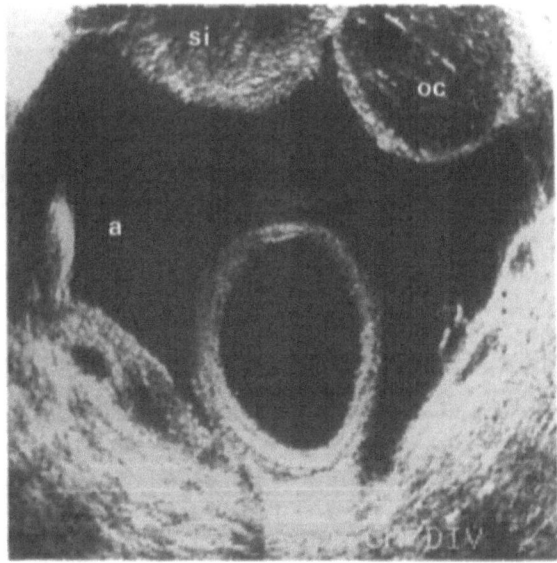

Fig. 7.8. Post-operative follow-up after anterior resection in a 40-year-old woman. Tumour stage at operation was uT3N1. The sonogram shows ascites (*a*). Further investigation revealed carcinomatosis of the peritoneum. *oc*, ovarian cyst; *si*, small intestine.

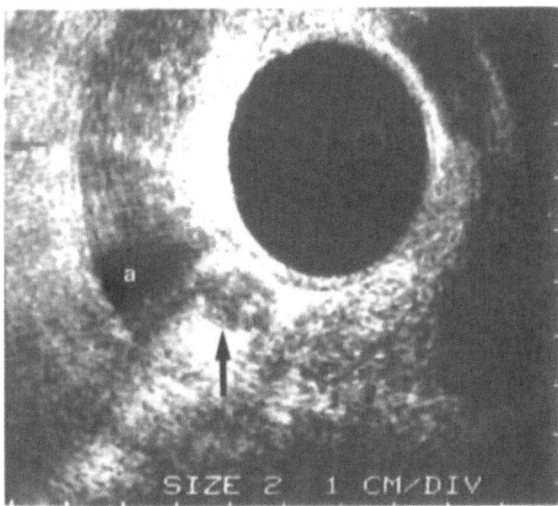

Fig. 7.9. An extrarectal recurrence in the 7 o'clock position (*arrow*). There was no mucosal evidence of recurrence and the diagnosis was confirmed by transperineal biopsy under ultrasound control. *a*, artefact.

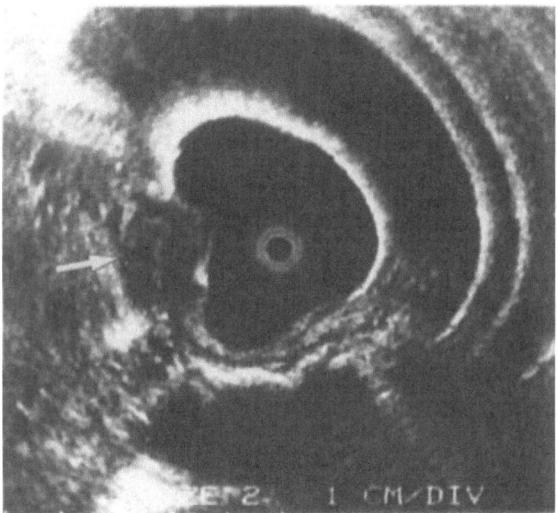

Fig. 7.10. In this case of recurrence, even though the tumour (*arrow*) does not involve the mucosa it is bulging into the rectal lumen.

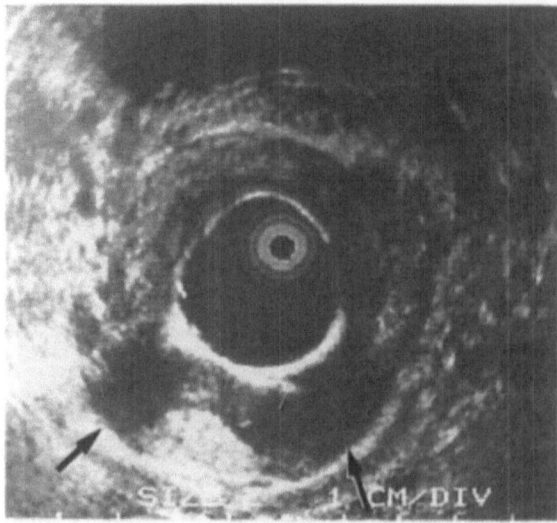

Fig. 7.11. This patient did not have any clinical evidence of recurrence. Ultrasonically, however, there was a large, mainly hypoechoic area surrounding the rectum which was recurrent tumour (*arrows*).

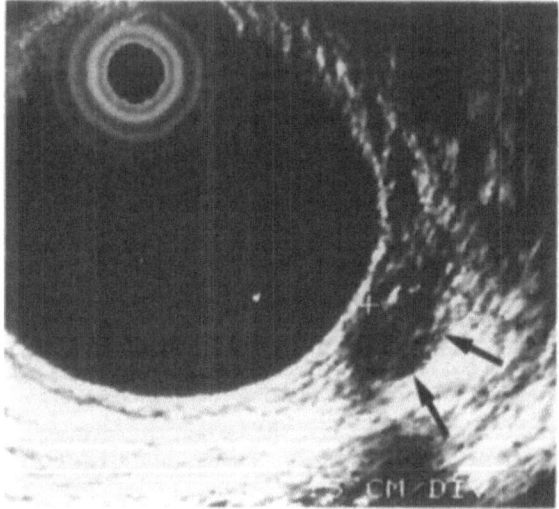

Fig. 7.12. Biopsy of the lesion seen enlarged here (*arrows*) failed to confirm the presence of recurrence. Subsequent scanning has shown no change in its size.

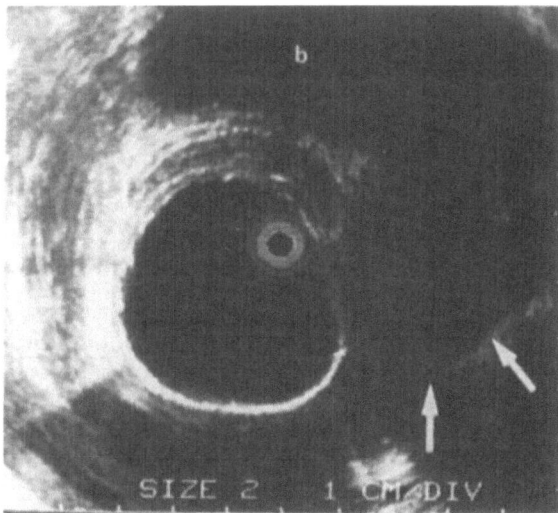

Fig. 7.13. This patient clinically had a palpable mass on the left side of the pelvis. Ultrasonically this was hypoechoic and circular (*arrows*). The bladder is seen anteriorly (*b*). Biopsy confirmed the presence of pus formed from a necrotic recurrent tumour.

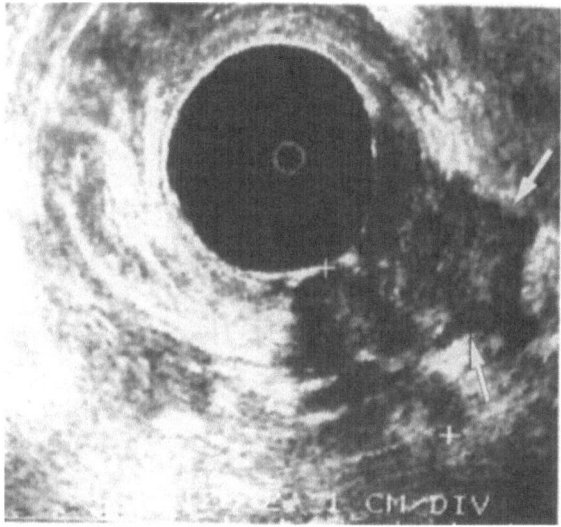

Fig. 7.14. A large recurrent rectal carcinoma (*arrows*).

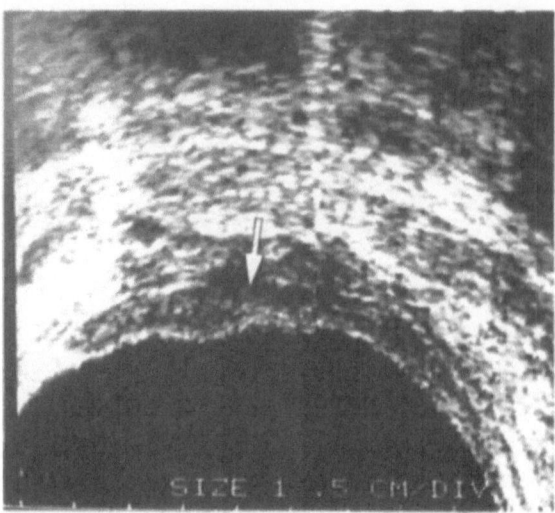

Fig. 7.15. This patient was treated by anterior resection for a primary rectal adenocarcinoma. Endosonographically there was a small hypoechoic area (*arrowed*) within the wall which had disrupted the layers. Full-thickness biopsy confirmed the presence of tumour, which was covered by granulation tissue on the luminal aspect.

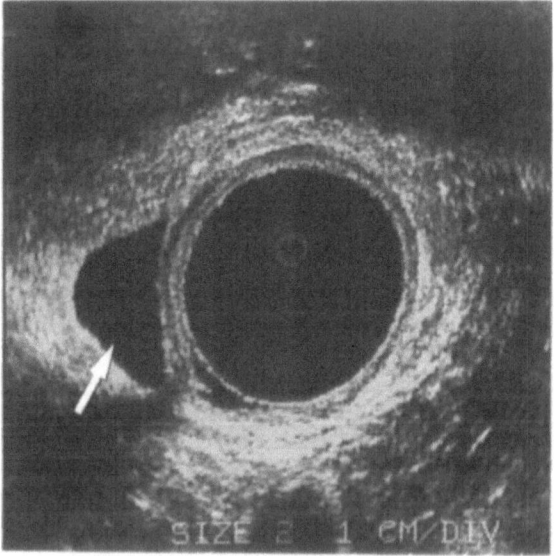

Fig. 7.16. Perirectal haematoma (*arrow*) following transperineal ultrasound-guided puncture of a dubious lesion.

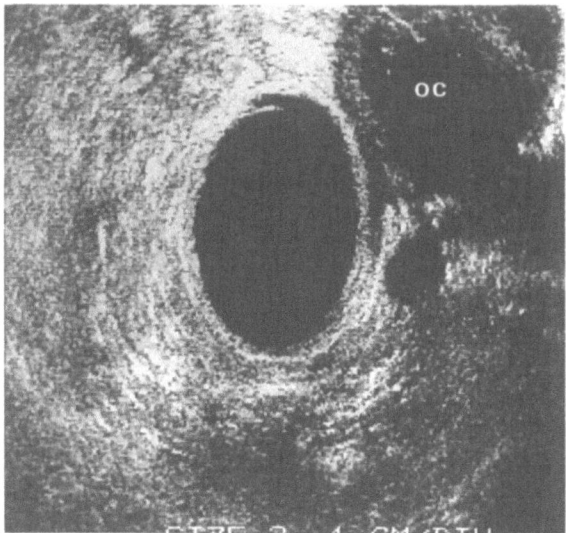

Fig. 7.17. Ovarian cyst (*oc*) seen during post-operative follow-up examination.

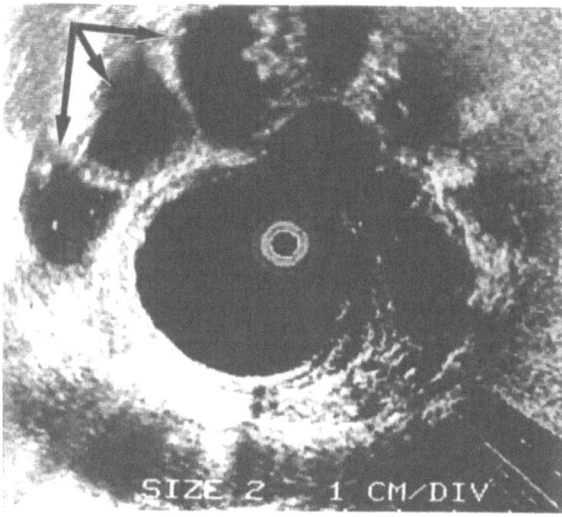

Fig. 7.18. Following surgery the anatomical relationships in the pelvis may be different, as illustrated by this scan of a patient following a "Hartmann" procedure. The endoprobe was introduced into the rectal stump and a large number of small bowel loops were imaged anteriorly (*arrows*).

8 Benign Rectal Tumours, Anal Canal, Perianal Disease and Other Conditions

Benign Rectal Tumours: Adenomas

Adenomas are divided into three categories histologically: tubular, tubulo-villous and villous. They can range in size from 1 mm to larger than 10 cm and be either pedunculated or sessile. Generally the larger the adenoma the greater the likelihood of a focus of malignant invasion. Polypoid adenomas smaller than 1 cm in diameter have less than a 1% incidence of invasion, whereas in adenomas larger than 2 cm there is a 35% incidence of invasion in polypoid lesions and 50% for flat villous adenomas. It is because of their malignant potential and the ensuing problems in surgical management that the endosonographic appearance of adenomas is so important.

Endosonographic Appearance (Figs. 8.1 to 8.6)

There are a number of technical problems in scanning adenomas. The water-filled balloon will squash and distort the anatomy of a polyp and care should be taken to reduce the volume in the balloon as much as possible. On some occasions it is helpful to fill the rectum with water first and use the minimum in the water balloon so as to distort the anatomy as little as possible. Very small lesions are easily missed and the endoprobe is best placed at the level of a small adenoma via a rectoscope, having first located it visually.

Adenomas have a hypoechoic appearance similar to that of invasive cancer but this is not uniform. Flat villous adenomas have a thickened inner hypoechoic layer representing the mucosa. Polypoid adenomas are divided into multiple nodules by clefts which can be pushed apart and flattened or layered by the water balloon. Air trapped between the water balloon and adenoma or rectal wall can give rise to artefacts. Malignant change and early invasion are very difficult to assess unless there is a sizeable uT1 tumour arising within an adenoma. Carcinoma in situ and severe dysplasia will clearly be impossible to detect.

Following excision biopsy of an invasive adenoma the rectum can be scanned for lymph nodes. The biopsy site will be distorted anatomically so that residual invasive tumour may also be difficult to assess. Repeated scanning at intervals may be useful.

In patients with ulcerative colitis complicated by a rectal villous adenoma or severe dysplasia the same reservations apply. The rectal wall and individual layers may be thickened, and inflammatory lymph nodes may give rise to some confusion when obvious cancers are assessed (Figs. 8.7 and 8.8).

Anal Canal and Perianal Disease

Despite the technical difficulty of inflating the water balloon in the anal canal and thus placing areas of interest within the focal range of the transducer, the anal canal can be scanned using either small volumes in the balloon or a special echolucent plastic cap over the transducer.

Sphincter Injuries

Traumatic injury to the anal sphincter results in partial or complete disruption of the external anal sphincter and occasionally the internal anal sphincter. Although there may be a cutaneous scar on clinical examination, the extent of the fibrous scar in the sphincter complex may be difficult to assess. Electromyographic (EMG) mapping with a needle is commonly used but can be painful for the patient. Early experience using anal ultrasound suggests that it may be as good as EMG (Fig. 8.9).

The scar has a hyperechoic appearance extending outwards radially. The thickness of the internal anal sphincter can also be assessed.

Perianal Abscess and Fistula (Fig. 8.10)

A fluid-filled abscess cavity is hypoechoic, and local anatomy is distorted by swelling and oedema. Endosonography can be especially helpful in patients where there is anal pain but little to see in the way of erythema or swelling, by establishing an early diagnosis.

A submucosal abscess arises in an infected anal gland and develops upwards, presenting with a mass in the upper anal canal. The mucosa is thickened on endosonography and the hypoechoic internal sphincter and hypoechoic abscess fuse together. The outermost interface shows a sharp demarcation of the perirectal fat.

An intersphincteric abscess will have the appearance of a hypoechoic mass which cannot be distinguished from the internal and external sphincter on either side of it.

A supralevator abscess outside the rectal wall will have the dark hypoechoic appearance of a water-filled cavity sometimes with inhomogeneous debris within it. The adjacent rectal wall is thickened and oedematous.

Fistula in ano can be demonstrated by anal endosonography. In order to show up the tracks, a solution of hydrogen peroxide is injected along the external opening. The resulting air bubbles help to delineate the fistula from surrounding structures. Where there is an associated chronic intersphincteric abscess it will have the features already described.

Anal Canal Tumours (Fig. 8.11 to 8.14)

Squamous or epidermoid and transitional cloacogenic carcinoma of the anal canal can be demonstrated by endosonography and depth of invasion can be assessed by disruption of the mucosa, internal and external sphincter. The tumours sited above the dentate line can metastasize to mesorectal lymph nodes, and endosonographic assessment of nodal involvement is very important. Since the introduction of chemotherapy and radiotherapy regimes for these tumours, an objective assessment of tumour response has been needed and endosonography has a role before and after treatment.

The Prostate (Fig. 8.15)

Although prostate ultrasound is not within the remit of this atlas, prostatic malignancy and abscess can give rise to diagnostic confusion. Advanced prostatic carcinoma can give the impression of an anterior rectal wall carcinoma, but endosonography will demonstrate its origin in the prostate, and the mucosal layer is usually intact. Smaller tumours of the prostate may be discovered coincidentally on rectal ultrasound. Prostatic abscess will give a heterogeneous hypoechoic pattern around the prostate gland area.

Other Rectal Tumours (Fig. 8.16 to 8.22)

Examples of scans of carcinoid tumour, leiomyosarcoma and lymphoma demonstrate that these do not have particular ultrasound features. Preservation of the mucosal layer will give some clue, and destruction of deeper layers and penetration into the surrounding mesorectum will indicate the extent of invasion.

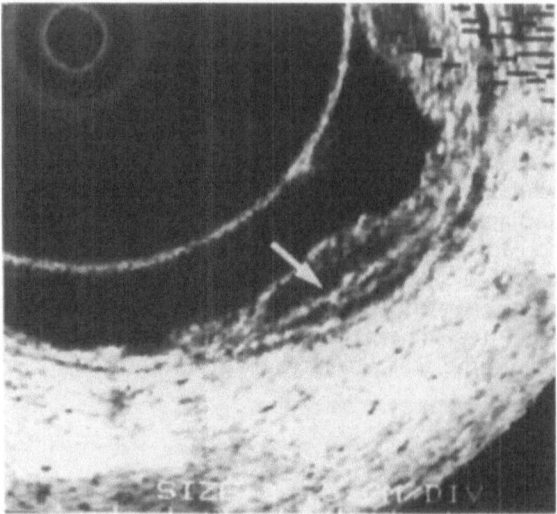

Fig. 8.1. An example of a large benign villous tumour. Note the "layering" of the squashed tumour (*arrow*).

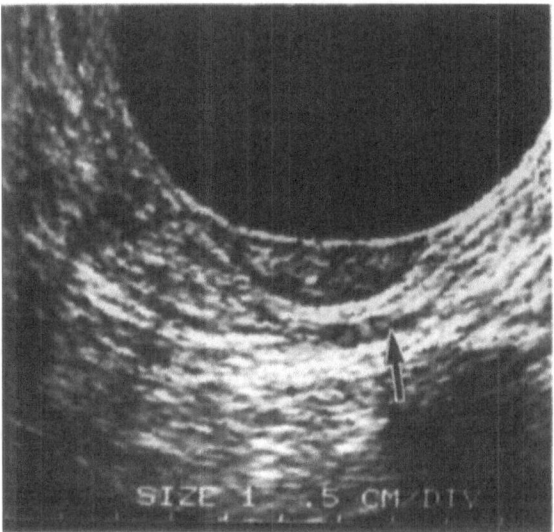

Fig. 8.2. Small adenoma. Note the intact outer layers (*arrow*).

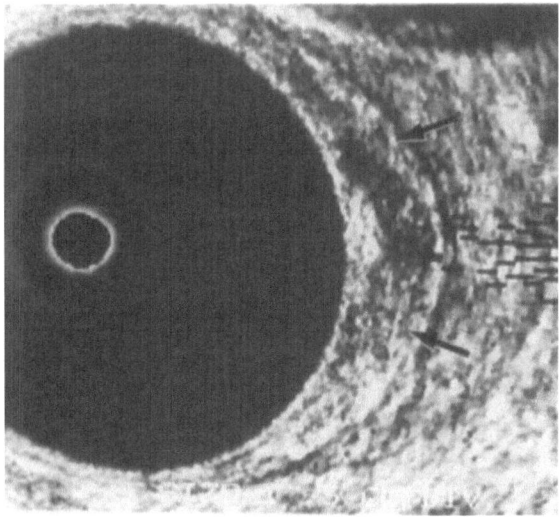

Fig. 8.3. This is another example of a large benign rectal tumour. The submucosal middle layer is clearly seen (*arrows*).

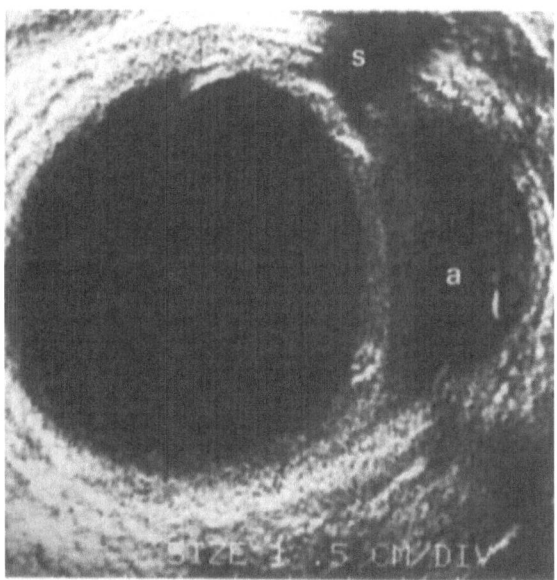

Fig. 8.4. Artefact: sonogram of an adenoma (*a*). The pedunculated adenoma is squeezed against the wall; an air bubble between water balloon and rectal wall and adenoma produces a shadow (*s*).

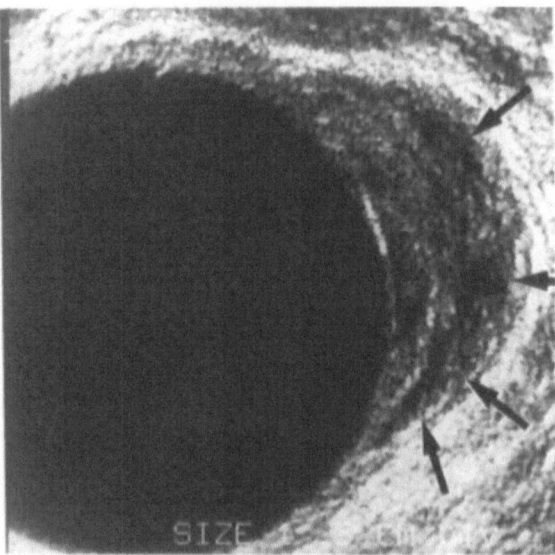

Fig. 8.5. Adenoma. The middle hyperechoic layer is seen along most of the edge (*arrows*).

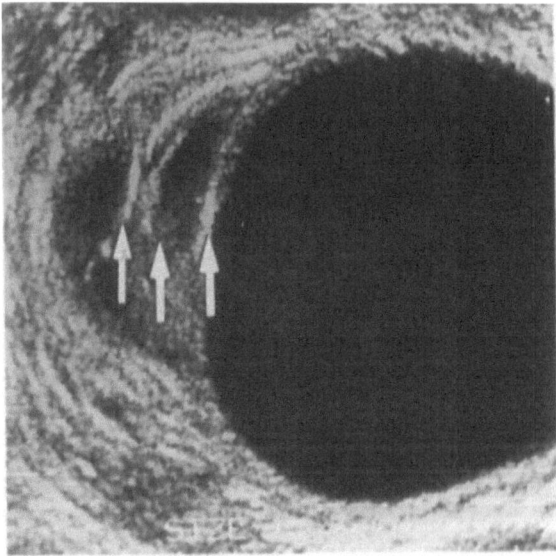

Fig. 8.6. Adenoma: inhomogeneous structure due to polypoid surface (*arrows*). Identification of a carcinoma in situ is not possible due to the inhomogeneous echogenicity of a benign lesion.

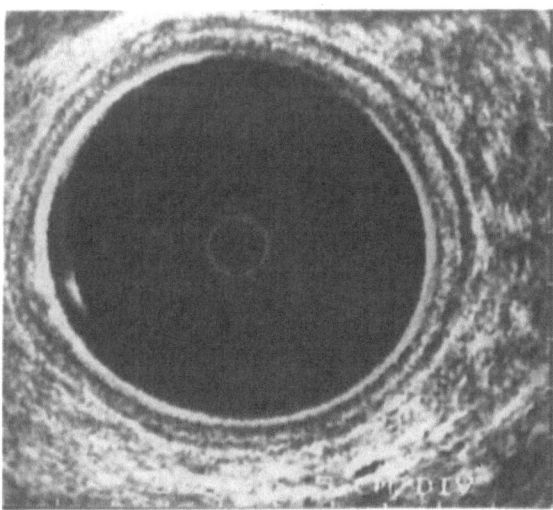

Fig. 8.7. An endosonogram of a patient with ulcerative colitis showing the five basic ultrasonic layers. There is nothing here to distinguish the sonogram from normal findings.

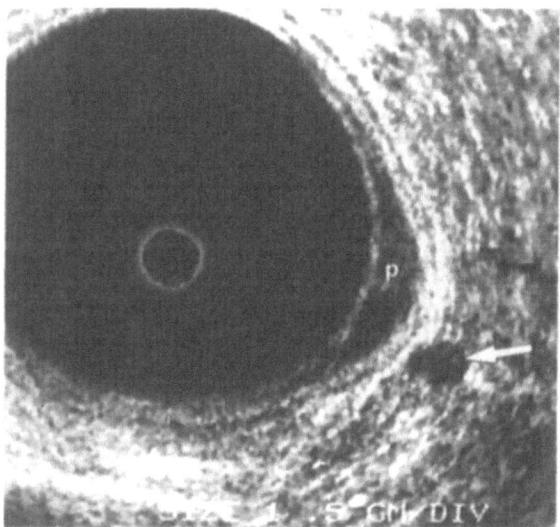

Fig. 8.8 A pseudopolyp (*p*) in a patient with marked ulcerative proctitis with an adjacent inflammatory node (*arrow*).

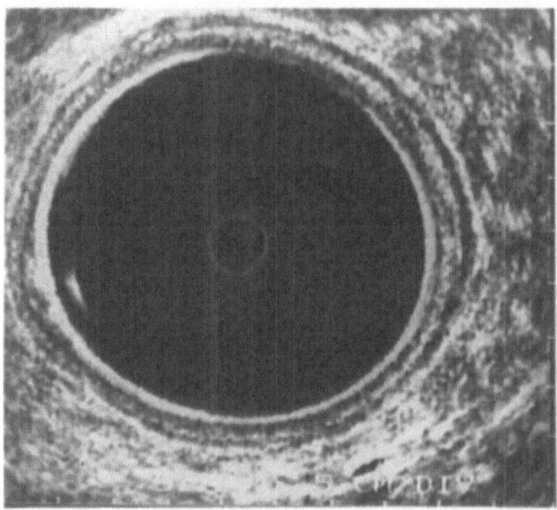

Fig. 8.9. Anal canal scan in a patient with an obstetric sphincter injury: *a*, anterior; *p*, posterior. The hypoechoic scar can be seen (*arrow*) between 9 o'clock and 12 o'clock.

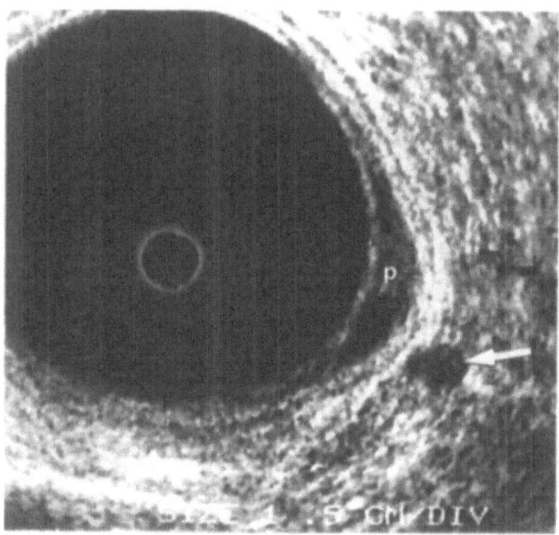

Fig. 8.10. Perianal abscess (*a*). *ias*, internal anal sphincter; *eas*, external anal sphincter.

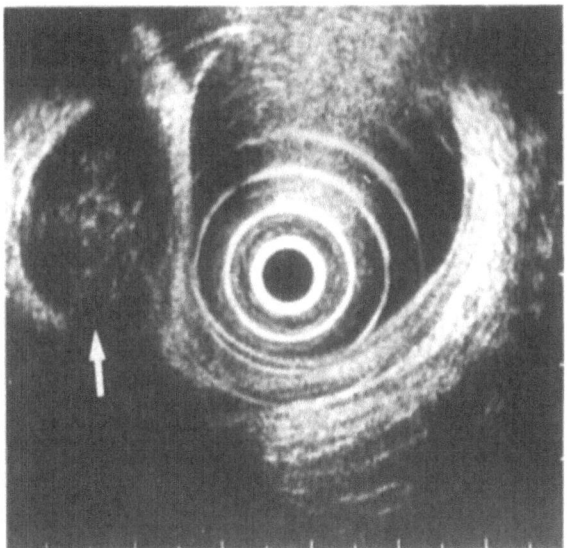

Fig. 8.11. With 12 MHz Olympus transducer. Within the outer hypoechoic layer there is an irregular mottled enlarged area – a leiomyoma of the muscularis propria (*arrowed*).

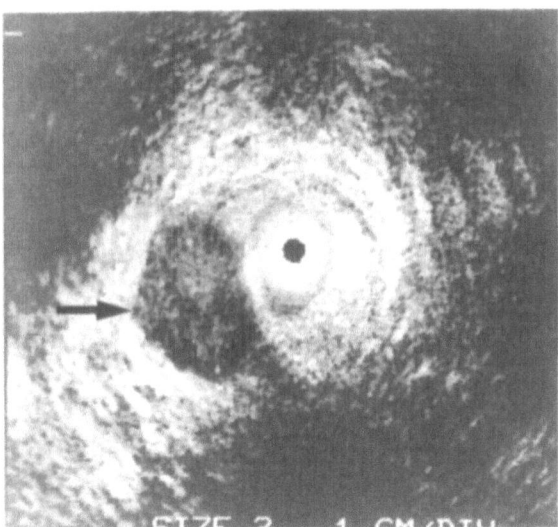

Fig. 8.12. Anal carcinoma (*arrow*).

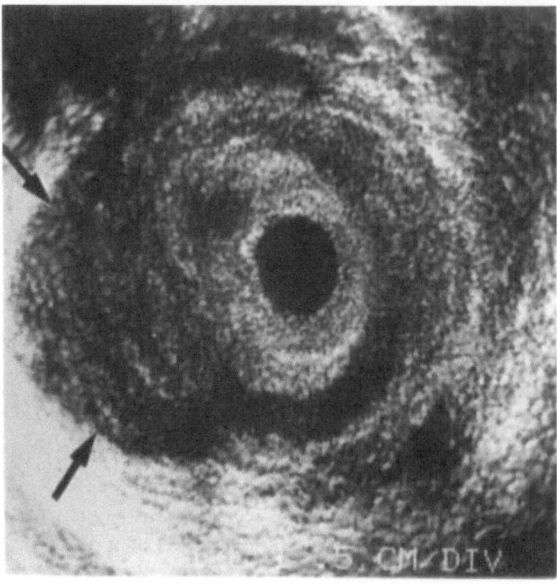

Fig. 8.13. Malignant melanoma of the anal canal (*arrows*) with penetration of the external anal sphincter but not perforation.

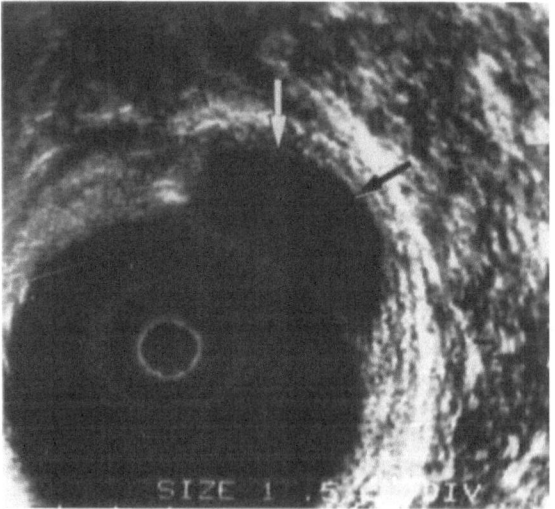

Fig. 8.14. This scan of a basaloid tumour has the same ultrasonic characteristics as the adenocarcinomas. The tumour here is confined by the submucosa (*arrows*).

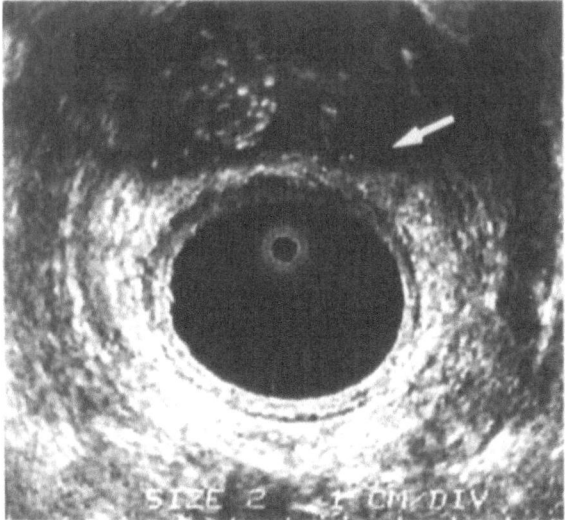

Fig. 8.15. A prostatic adenocarcinoma (*arrowed*).

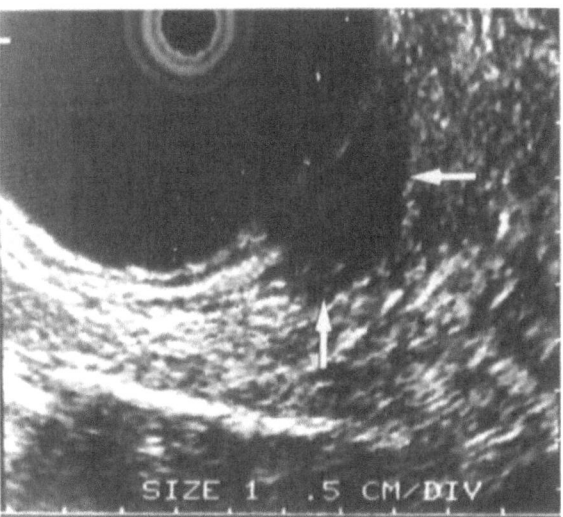

Fig. 8.16. A carcinoid tumour of the rectum (*arrow*). This is invading through all the layers of the rectal wall.

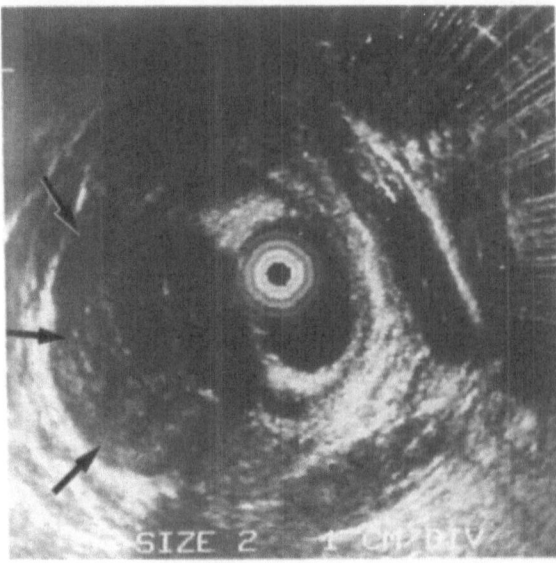

Fig. 8.17. A leiomyosarcoma of the rectum extending out to the pelvic side wall on the right side of the patient (*arrows*).

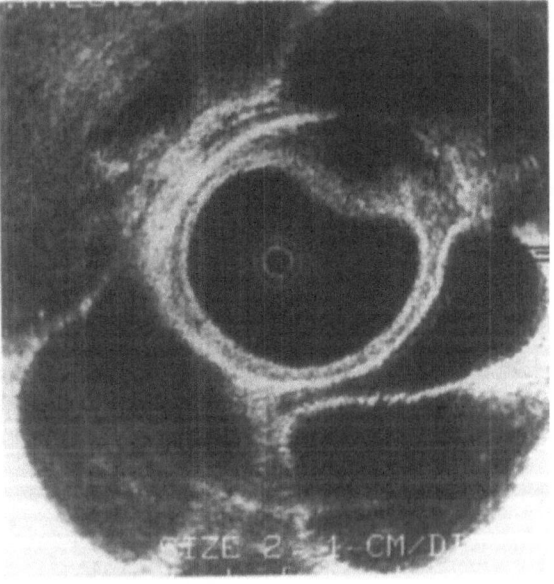

Fig. 8.18. Large ovarian cyst multilobular surrounding the rectum. Impression at anterior side.

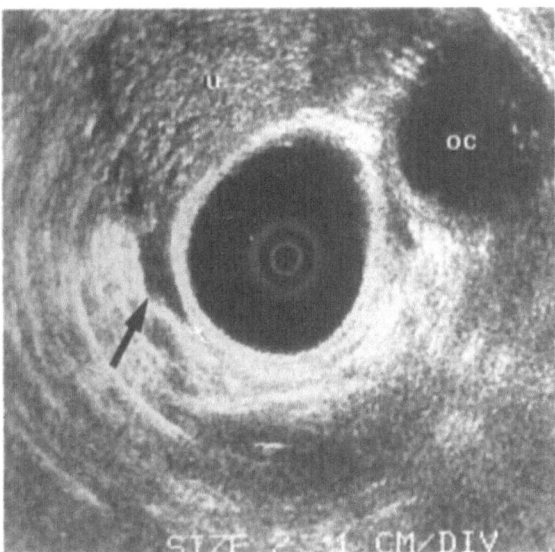

Fig. 8.19. Sonogram of a 27-year-old woman with endometriosis (*arrow*). *u*, uterus; *oc*, ovarian cyst.

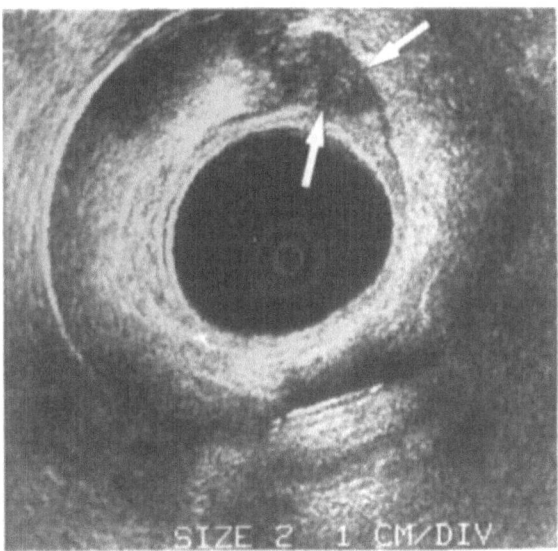

Fig. 8.20. Same patient as in Fig. 8.19, showing an area of infiltration of endometriosis into the muscularis of the rectal wall. The mucosa is intact (*arrows*).

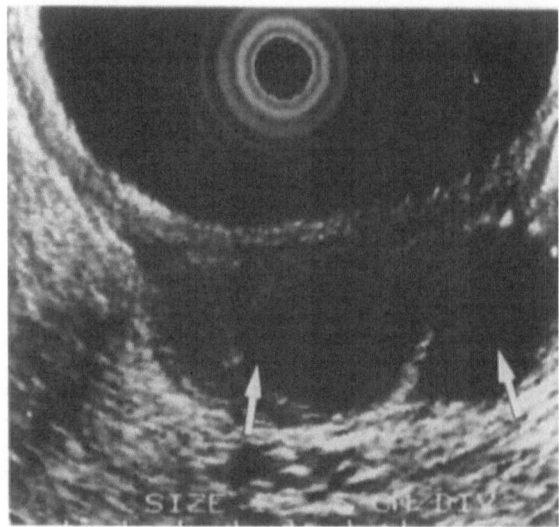

Fig. 8.21. A sonogram of a patient with a rectal re-
duplication. Small cystic areas are clearly seen behind the
rectum (*arrows*).

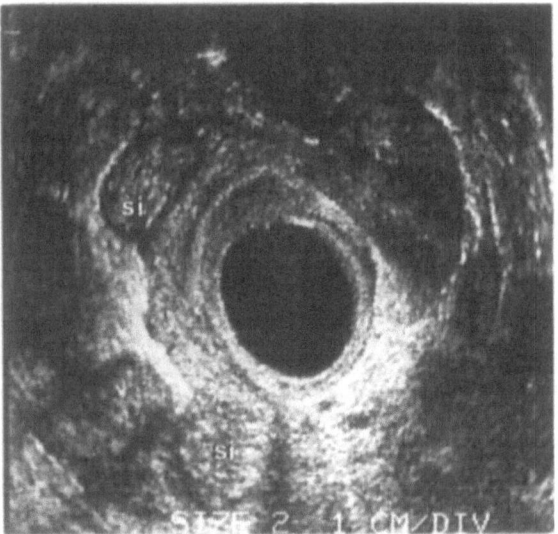

Fig. 8.22. Small intestine (*si*) loops around the rectum in
an elderly woman with rectal prolapse.

Appendix. TNM and pTNM Classification of Colorectal Carcinoma (From UICC, 1987, with permission)

TNM Clinical classification

T-primary tumour

TX Primary tumour cannot be assessed
TO No evidence of primary tumour
Tis Carcinoma in situ
T1 Tumour invades submucosa
T2 Tumour invades muscularis propria
T3 Tumour invades through muscularis propria into subserosa or into non-peritoneaslised pericolic or perirectal tissues
T4 Tumour perforates the visceral peritoneum or directly invades other organs or structures
Note: Direct invasion in T4 includes invasion of other segments of the colorectum by way of the serosa, e.g. invasion of the sigmoid colon by a carcinoma of the caecum.

N-regional lymph nodes

NX Regional lymph nodes cannot be assessed
NO No regional lymph node metastasis
N1 Metastasis in one to three pericolic or perirectal lymph nodes

N2 Metastasis in four or more pericolic or perirectal lymph nodes

N3 Metastasis in any lymph node along the course of a named vascular trunk

Note: The regional lymph nodes are the pericolic and perirectal and those located along the ileocolic, right colic, middle colic, left colic, inferior mesenteric and superior rectal (haemorrhoidal) arteries.

M-distant metastasis

MX Presence of distant metastasis cannot be assessed

MO No distant metastasis

M1 Distant metastasis

pTNM pathological classification

The pT, pN and pM categories correspond to the T, N and M categories

Bibliography

Adelsteinsson B, Glimelius B, Graffman S, Hemingsson A, Pahlman L (1985) Computed tomography in staging of rectal carcinoma. Acta Radiol [Diagn] 26: 45–55

Aibe T (1984a) A study on the structure of layers of the gastointestinal wall visualised by means of the ultrasonic endoscope. I. The structure of layers of the gastric wall. Gastroenterol Endosc 26: 1447–1464

Aibe T (1984b) A study on the structure of layers of the gastrointestinal wall visualised by means of the ultrasonic endoscope. II. The structure of layers of the esophageal wall and the colonic wall. Gastroenterol Endosc 26: 1465–1473

Alzin HH, Kohlberger E, Schwaiger R, Alloussi S (1983) Valeur de l'échographie endorectale dans la chirurgie du rectum. Ann Radiol 26: 334–336.

Beynon J (1989) An evaluation of the role of rectal endosonography in rectal cancer. Ann R Coll Surg Eng 71: 131–139

Beynon J, Mortensen NJMcC (1988) Staging rectal cancer with endosonography. Hosp Update 14: 1748–1754

Beynon J, Mortensen NJMcC (1989) Rectal endosonography in the pre-operative staging and follow-up of rectal cancer. Intern Med Specialist 10: 79–98

Beynon J, Foy DMA, Channer, JL, Temple LN, Virjee J, Mortensen NJMcC (1986a) The endosonic appearances of normal colon and rectum. Dis Colon Rectum 29: 810–813

Beynon J, Mortensen NJMcC, Foy DMA, Channer JL, Virjee J, Goddard P (1986b) Endorectal sonography: laboratory and clinical experience in Bristol. Int J Colorect Dis 1: 212–215

Beynon J, Mortensen NJMcC, Foy DMA, Channer JL, Virjee, J, Goddard P (1986c) Pre-operative assessment of local invasion in rectal cancer: digital examination, endoluminal sonography or computed tomography. Br J Surg 73: 1015–1017

Beynon J, Roe AM, Foy DMA, Channer JL, Virjee J, Mortensen NJMcC (1986d) Transrectal ultrasound or computed tomography for the assessment of local invasion in rectal cancer. Surg Forum 37: 199–201

Beynon J, Roe AM, Foy DMA, Temple LN, Mortensen NJMcC (1986e) Endoluminal ultrasound in the assessment of local invasion in rectal cancer. Br J Surg 73: 474–477

Beynon J, Mortensen NJMcC, Foy DMA, Channer JL, Virjee J, Goddard P (1987a) The radiological staging of rectal cancer. Coloproctology 9: 274–276

Beynon J, Roe AM. Foy DMA, Channer JL, Virjee J, Mortensen NJMcC (1987b) Pre-operative staging of local invasion in rectal cancer using endoluminal ultrasound. J R Soc Med 80: 23–24

Beynon J, Mortensen NJMcC, Rigby H (1988) Rectal endosonography: a new technique for the pre-operative staging of rectal cancer. Eur J Surg Oncol 14: 297–309

Beynon J, Mortensen NJMcC, Foy DMA, Channer JL, Rigby HS, Virjee J (1989a) Pre-operative assessment of meso-rectal lymph node involvement in rectal cancer. Br J Surg 76: 276–279

Beynon J, Mortensen NJMcC, Foy DMA, Rigby HS, Channer JL, Virjee J (1989b) The detection and evaluation of locally recurrent rectal cancer with rectal endosonography. Dis Colon Rectum 32: 509–517

Boscani M (1989) Lower gastrointestinal ultrasound. Surg Endosc 3: 29–32

Boscani M, Masoni L, Montori A (1986) Transrectal ultrasonography: three years' experience. Int J Colorectal Dis 1: 208–211

Butch RJ, Stark DD, Wittenburg J, Tepper JE, Saini S, Simeone JF, Mueller PR, Ferrucci JT (1986) Staging rectal cancer by MR and CT. Am J Radiol 146: 1155–1160

Caletti G, Bolondi L, Labo G (1984a) Anatomical aspects in ultrasonic endoscopy of the stomach. Scand J Gastroentrol 19 [Suppl 94]: 34–42

Caletti G, Bolondi L, Labo G (1984b) Ultrasonic endoscopy: the gastrointestinal wall. Scand J Gastroenterol 19 [Suppl 102]: 5–8

Cooper A, Edwards SF (1892) Diseases of rectum and anus, 2nd edit. J & A Churchill, London

Dimagno EP, Regan PT, Clain JE, James EM, Buxton JL (1982) Human endoscopic ultrasonography. Gastroenterology 83: 824–829

Dixon AK, Fry IK, Morson BC, Nicholls RJ, York Mason A (1981) Pre-operative computed tomography of carcinoma of the rectum. Br J Radiol 54: 655–659

Dragstedt J, Gammelgaard J (1983) Endoluminal ultrasonic scanning in the evaluation of rectal cancer. Gastrointest Radiol 8: 367–369

Feifel G, Hildebrandt U, Koch B, Alzin H (1984) The ultrasonic imaging of the rectum. In: Givel JC, Saegesser F (eds) Coloproctology. Springer, Berlin Heidelberg New York, pp. 3–8

Feifel G, Hildebrandt U, Dhom G (1985) Die endorektale Sonographie beim Rektumcarcinom. Chirurgie 56: 398–402

Feifel G, Hildebrandt U, Mortensen NJMcC (eds) (1990) Endosonography in Gastroenterology, Gynaecology and Urology. Springer, Berlin Heidelberg New York.

Freeny PC, Feldberg MAM, Van Waes PFGM (1986) Preoperative staging of rectal cancer with computerized tomography: accuracy, efficacy and effect on patient management. Radiology 158: 347–353

Fukuda M (1985) Endoscopic ultrasonography. In: Proceedings of the World Federation of Ultrasound in Medicine and Biology, pp. 13–16 (Abstr)

Grabbe E, Lierse W, Winkler R (1983) The perirectal fascia: morphology and use in staging of rectal carcinoma. Radiology 149: 241–246

Hamlin DJ, Burgener FA, Sischy B (1981) New technique to stage early rectal carcinoma by computed tomography. Radiology 141: 539–540.

Hildebrandt U, Feifel G (1985) Pre-operative staging of rectal cancer by intrarectal ultrasound. Dis Col Rectum 28: 42–46

Hildebrandt U, Feifel G (1986) Endosonographische Bestimmung der Infiltrationstiefe und Beurteilung von Lymphknoten beim Rektumkarzinom. Ultraschall Klin Prax 1: 89–94

Hildebrandt U, Feifel G, Schwarz HP, Scherr O (1986) Endorectal ultrasound: instrumentation and clinical aspects. Int J Colorectal Dis 1: 203–207

Hodgman CG, MacCarty RL, Wolff BG, May GR, Berquist TH, Sheedy PF, Beart RW, Spencer RJ (1986) Pre-operative staging of rectal carcinoma by computed tomography and 0.15T magnetic resonance imaging. Dis Colon Rectum 29: 446–450

Holdsworth PJ, Johnston D, Chalmers AG, Chennells P, Dixon MF, Finan PF, Primrose JN, Quirke P (1988) Endoluminal ultrasound and computed tomography in the staging of rectal cancer. Br J Surg 75: 1019–1022

Johnson RJ, Jenkins JPR, Isherwood I (1987a) Magnetic resonance imaging in oncology. In: Bleehen N (ed) Investigational techniques in oncology. Springer, Berlin Heidelberg New York, pp. 125–151

Johnson RJ, Jenkins JPR, Isherwood I, James RD, Schofield PF, (1987b) Quantative magnetic resonance imaging in rectal cancer. Br J Radiol 60: 761–764

Law PJ, Talbot RW, Bartram CI, Northover JMA (1989) Anal endosonography in the evaluation of perianal sepsis and fistula in ano. Br J Surg 76: 752–755

Konishi F, Muto T, Takahashi H, Itoh K, Kanazawa K. Morioka Y (1985) Transrectal ultrasonography for the assessment of invasion of rectal carcinoma. Dis Colon Rectum 28: 889–894

Kramann B, Hildebrandt U (1986) Computed tomography versus endosonography in the staging of rectal carcinoma: a comparative study. Int J Colorectal Dis 1: 216–218

Kumegawa H, Murata Y, Akimoto S, Yoshida M, Endo M (1985) Study of endoscopic ultrasonography for esophageal carcimoma. Jpn J Med Ultrasonics 12: 21–28

Masgagni D, Corbellini L, Urciuoli P, Matteo G (1989) Endoluminal ultrasound for the detection of local recurrence in rectal cancer. Br J Surg 76: 1176–1180

Nicholls RJ, York Mason A, Morson BC, Dixon AK, Kelsey Fry I (1982) The clinical staging of rectal cancer. Br J Surg 69: 404–409

Rifkin MD, Marks GJ (1985) Transrectal US as an adjunct in the diagnosis of rectal and extrarectal tumours. Radiology 157: 499–502

Rifkin MD, Wechsler RJ (1986) A comparison of computed tomography and endorectal ultrasound in staging rectal cancer. Int J Colorectal Dis 1: 219–223

Romano G, De Rosa P, Vallone G, Rotondo A, Grassi R, Saint Angelo ML (1985) Intrarectal ultrasound and computed tomography in the pre- and post-operative assessment of patients with rectal carcinoma. Br J Surg 72 [suppl]: S117–S119

Saitoh N, Okui K, Sarashina H, Suzuki M, Arai T, Nanomura M (1986) Evaluation of echographic diagnosis of rectal cancer using intrarectal ultrasonic examination. Dis Colon Rectum 29: 234–242

Sobin LH, Hermanek P, Hutter RVP (1988) TNM classification of malignant tumours. A comparison between the new (1987) and the old editions. Cancer 61: 2310–2314

Thoeni RF, Moss AA, Schneyder T, Margulis AR (1981) Detection and staging of primary rectal and rectosigmoid cancer by computed tomography. Radiology 141: 135–138

Thompson LM, Calvorsen RA (1987) Computed tomographic staging of gastrointestinal malignancies. Part I. The small bowel, colon and rectum. J Invest Radiol 22 (2): 96–105

Thompson WM, Calvorsen RA, Foster WL, Roberts L, Gibbon R (1986) Pre-operative and postoperative CT staging of rectosigmoid carcinoma. Am J Radiol 146: 703–710

Tio TL, Tygat GN (1984) Endoscopic ultrasonography in the assessment of intra- and transmural infiltration of tumours in the oesophagus, stomach and papilla of Vater and in the detection of extraoesophageal lesions. Endoscope 16: 203–210

UICC (1987) Hermanek P, Sobin LH (eds) TNM classification of malignant tumours, 4th edn. Springer, Berlin Heidelberg New York

Van Waes PFGM, Koehler PR, Feldberg NAM (1983) Management of rectal carcinoma: impact of computed tomography. Am J Radiol 140: 1137–1142

Watanabe H (1979) Prostatic ultrasound. In: Rosenfield AT (ed) Genitourinary ultrasonography. Churchill Livingstone, London, pp. 125–137

Wild JJ (1950) The use of ultrasonic pulses for the measurement of biologic tissues and the detection of tissue density changes. Surgery 27: 183–188

Wild JJ, Foderick JW (1978a) The feasibility of echometric detection of cancer in the lower gastrointestinal tract. I. Am J Proct, Gastro Col, Rectal Surg [Jan–Feb]: 16–25

Wild JJ, Foderick JW (1978b) The feasibility of echometric detection of cancer of the lower gastrointestinal tract. II. Am J Proct Gastro Col, Rectal Surg [Mar–Apr]: 11–20

Wild JJ, Reid JM (1952) Further pilot echographic studies of the histologic structure of tumours of the living intact human breast. Am J Pathol 28: 839–854

Wild JJ, Reid JM (1956) Diagnostic use of ultrasound. Br J Phys Med 19: 248–257

Yamashita Y, Machi J, Shirouzu K, Morotomi T, Isomoto H, Kakegawa T (1988) Evaluation of endorectal ultrasound for the assessment of wall invasion of rectal cancer. Dis Colon Rectum 31: 617–623

Yashuda K, Tanaka Y, Fujimoto S, Makajima M, Kawai K (1984) Use of endoscopic ultrasonography in small pancreatic cancer. Scand J Gastroenterol 19 [Suppl 102]: 9–17

Yorke-Mason A (1976) Rectal cancer: the spectrum of selective surgery. Proc R Soc Med 69: 237–244

Zaunbauer W, Haertel M, Fuchs WA (1981) Computed tomography in carcinoma of the rectum. Gastrointest Radiol 6: 79–84

Zelas P, Haaga JR, Lavery IC, Fazio VW (1980) The diagnosis by percutaneous biopsy with computed tomography of a recurrence of carcinoma of the rectum in the pelvis. Surg Gynecol Obstet 151: 525–527

Zheng G, Eddleston B, Schofield PF, Johnson RJ, James RD (1984) Computed tomographic scanning in rectal cancer. J R Soc Med 77: 915–920